MW00941450

Shaken Baby Syndrome or Vaccine Induced Encephalitis - Are Parents Being Falsely Accused?

Harold Buttram M.D.
and
Christina England, Research Journalist

authorHOUSE®

AuthorHouse™
1663 Liberty Drive
Bloomington, IN 47403
www.authorhouse.com
Phone: 1-800-839-8640

© 2011 Harold Buttram M.D. and Christina England. All rights reserved.

No part of this book may be reproduced, stored in a retrieval system, or transmitted by any means without the written permission of the author.

First published by AuthorHouse 2/8/2011

ISBN: 978-1-4567-1975-3 (dj)
ISBN: 978-1-4567-1974-6 (e)
ISBN: 978-1-4567-1976-0 (sc)

Library of Congress Control Number: 2011900294

Printed in the United States of America

Any people depicted in stock imagery provided by Thinkstock are models, and such images are being used for illustrative purposes only. Certain stock imagery © Thinkstock.

This book is printed on acid-free paper.

Because of the dynamic nature of the Internet, any Web addresses or links contained in this book may have changed since publication and may no longer be valid. The views expressed in this work are solely those of the author and do not necessarily reflect the views of the publisher, and the publisher hereby disclaims any responsibility for them.

Designer Peter Irvin of - Old School Computer Training www.osct.co.uk

Contents

Acronyms:

SBS: Shaken Baby Syndrome
NAI: Non-Accidental Trauma
LMF: Lethal Minor Fall
SIS: Sudden Impact Syndrome
AHT: Abusive Head Trauma
SIDS: Sudden Infant Death Syndrome
DAI: Diffuse Axonal Injury

Dedications

H. Buttram

This book is dedicated to those biomechanicians whose research work, though not yet fully appreciated, has totally disproved and falsified the *Shaken Baby Syndrome theory*; to a small group of forensic pathologists and other physicians who have been actively defending parents and caretakers accused of this syndrome; and to falsely accused parents and caretakers whose lives have been devastated. It is also dedicated to those infants and children who have been removed from their parents and placed in foster homes, something that will come to be looked upon as *legalized kidnapping* in future and wiser times.

Christina England

I dedicate this book to.....

All of the parents who have been falsely accused of shaken baby syndrome after their child has suffered an adverse reaction to a vaccine. I hope that this book goes a long way toward helping you prove your innocence and get justice and peace in your life. May this book open the world's eyes to a differential diagnosis to that of Shaken Baby Syndrome and steer professionals toward investigating all avenues of possibility before blaming what could potentially be innocent parents.

My two beautiful children, Daniel and Nicholas England, who have helped me to understand autism and have brought so much joy into my life. I am so very proud of you both.

My late parents, Joan and Norman England, who were there for me and who supported me when I was falsely accused of Munchausen by proxy. May you rest in peace.

My brother Graham and his family, who have supported me through some very difficult times, always trying to understand and be there not only for myself but for my two children.

Gary and Lyn Cox, who have been amazing friends and neighbors, especially Gary, who is always at hand to help me survive computer technology. My friend Edna Franklin, who I meet for coffee most mornings. Leslie Botha, Jeffry Aufderheide, Clifford Miller, and Dr. Michael Innis, all professionals who have believed in me. Zabeth Bayne, a falsely accused parent herself, who has made this book possible while suffering the pain of having her beautiful children taken from her. And, of course, Dr. Harold Buttram, who asked me to be his coauthor. Thank you all so very much.

I would especially like to thank one friend and professional in particular, psychologist and expert in autism Lisa Blakemore-Brown, who gave me back my self-belief. Without her, I would never have been able to contribute to this book. She has been an amazing inspiration in my life. She believed everything I said when I was falsely accused, being forever supportive and encouraging. She has been my shining light through some very dark days. She has opened my eyes up to the possibility that vaccines can have adverse reactions and has taught me so much about autistic spectrum disorders and how to help my children. Despite all her problems, she has continued to speak out and help children with autism worldwide. I owe you so much, Lisa. Thank you; please keep fighting. You are truly a special friend in my life.

I would also like to mention the many other friends and colleagues around the world who read my work and encourage me to write. Thank you.

Finally I would like to dedicate this book to Cameron Bruce, a premature baby who sadly died at the tender age of two months, leaving behind his twin brother, Dalton, and Mike and Elizabeth, his dedicated parents, who were falsely accused and cleared of shaken baby syndrome.

May God bless you all.

Introduction

Shaken Baby Syndrome (SBS)/Non-Accidental Injury (NAI) cases fall in three general categories:

(1) *Shaken Baby Syndrome,* (SBS) in which it is assumed that a parent or caretaker, irritated and exhausted by a fussy baby, picks up the infant by his or her chest and shakes the baby with such violence that any onlooker would recognize it as excessive and dangerous. In hospitals throughout the U.S.A it is assumed that if an infant is brought into the emergency department with findings of brain and/or retinal hemorrhages without known history of a major impact such as auto accident or high distance fall, it is assumed that the infant had been subjected to the SBS and/or NAI.

(2) *Non-Accidental Trauma* (NAT) in which it is assumed there may be incidental impact of head, limbs, or body against a solid object during the shaking, or from direct blows inflicted by the caretaker.

(3) *Infants with multiple fractures,* which is dealt with in a separate monograph, available on request from the author.

Based on personal observations of more than 10 years in each of these categories, there have often been patterns of precipitous diagnoses of inflicted child abuse without first establishing a reasonably thorough differential diagnosis and ruling out other possible causes of the findings.

Due to these deficiencies in differential diagnoses, in my opinion, many parents and caretakers are being falsely accused and criminally convicted; children are unjustly being removed from their parents and placed in foster homes. In any other medical specialty, these failures to establish a differential diagnosis of the findings would be considered substandard and unacceptable medical practice. This statement is based on long-established medical traditions dating back to Sir William Osler (1849-1919), generally considered to be the father of internal medicine and the art of medical diagnosis.

This paper also challenges current childhood vaccine programs, an area generally considered sacrosanct, as the true source of many brain and retinal hemorrhages that are being misdiagnosed as Shaken Baby Syndrome and/or Inflicted Child Abuse. This is largely based on the principle that combinations of toxic chemicals may bring exponential increases in toxicity; that is, two toxic chemicals in combination may bring a ten-fold or even an hundred-fold increase in toxicity. In vaccines, these chemicals would be mercury, aluminum, formaldehyde, antibiotics, and others. This principle was originally established by the classic experiment of J Schubert *et al* (*Journal of Toxicology and Environmental Health,* 1978) in which it was found that doses of the neurotoxic metals, lead and mercury, when injected separately into rats, caused *one percent fatalities* (LD1), but when injected in combination caused *one hundred percent fatalities* (LD100) (1). Since that time others have confirmed this same principle under a variety of circumstances (2-4). This subject will be reviewed in some depth in chapter 7 on the "five-in-one vaccines" by Christina England.

Chapter 1

The Alleged Shaken
Baby Syndrome

(A) Origin of the Shaken Baby Syndrome (SBS)

Working with the U.S. Department of Transportation, an Oxford-trained neurosurgeon, AK Ommaya, devised an experiment to measure the amount of rotational acceleration required to reach the threshold of brain injury with adult Rhesus monkeys as subjects. As reviewed by R Uscinski:

> "A contoured fiberglass chair was built, mounted on wheels, and placed on tracks with a piston behind it. The monkeys were strapped into the chair with their heads free to rotate in such a way that there would be no impact. The piston then impacted the chair, simulating a rear-end motor vehicle collision. The experiment was photographed with a high-speed camera, allowing calculations of generated rotational accelerations. Ommaya was able to demonstrate that a rotational acceleration of 40,000 radians/second (squared) was sufficient to produce intracranial injury in 19 of the animals, with 11 (57.9%) of them also demonstrating neck injuries. Then, using the scaling parameters, he estimated that less rotational acceleration would be required to produce concussion in the larger human brain, perhaps on the order of 6,000 to 7,000 radians/second (squared)"(5).

1

Calculations were based on the same laws as described in classical Newtonian physics, as applied to movements of planetary bodies, that force is the product of mass and acceleration.

Ommaya's experiments were published in the *Journal of the American Medical Association* in 1968 (6). In 1971 Guthkelch reported on the first diagnosed case of SBS in which he hypothesized that subdural hematomas could be caused by manually shaking an infant without the head impacting on any surface (7). One year later Caffey, a radiologist, alluded to the parent-infant stress syndrome with manual shaking causing intracranial injury in the form of subdural hematoma and/or retinal hemorrhages of infants. (8) Two additional papers published by Caffey over the next two years emphasized shaking as a means of inflicting intracranial bleeding in children (9,10). It is important to note that each of these four papers referred to Ommaya's publication of 1968 as justification for this concept. This was in spite of the fact that Caffey, in a phone consultation with Ommaya, had been assured by Ommaya that his monkey tests could not be used to support the SBS hypothesis.

After publication of these four papers, the term Shaken Baby Syndrome became widely accepted as a clinical diagnosis for inflicted (non-accidental) head injury in infants in which the findings of subdural (brain) hemorrhages and/or retinal hemorrhages became accepted as exclusively diagnostic of SBS in the absence of known major accidental trauma and remains so today in hospital emergency rooms..

(B) SBS Theory Irreconcilable with the Weakness of the Human Infant's Neck

From its origins, the SBS has been based on the assumption that a parent or caretaker, becoming irritated over a baby's prolonged fussiness and crying, loses self-control and, grasping the infant by the chest or heels, shakes the infant with such violence that any onlooker would recognize it as excessive and dangerous. It is true that shaking does sometimes take place when an infant collapses and stops breathing, which is a common presentation in many of these cases. In such situations a panicky parent, usually untrained in resuscitation, may pick up an infant and (not knowing what else to do) **mildly** shakes an infant that has just gone into respiratory arrest. However, these instances **do not** in any sense constitute SBS.

As pointed out in the Uscinski report (5). the brain of an infant is nearly seven times larger and heavier than that of a monkey. In addition, adult monkeys are known to be incredibly strong, approximately four times stronger than humans. There would be no comparison, therefore, between the neck muscle strength of an adult monkey and that of an infant, barely able to hold up his or her head by age six months. Consequently, if such violent shaking were actually taking place, It follows that the incidence of neck injuries in the SBS should be exponentially greater than the 59.7 percent in Ommaya's monkey experiment. With these facts in mind, consider the following:

'Most SBS cases in the USA take place during the first six months of life, when there are negligible infant neck muscles. As will be shown further on, the major impact of violent shaking would fall at the junction between the base of the skull and brainstem area and upper cervical spinal cord. In most if not all instances this would result in instant death or paraplegia (spinal paralysis) from brain stem and/or cervical spinal cord injuries.

'Biomechanical research literature consistently reports findings that infant subdural hemorrhages in a 2-yr.-old child can not take place below a range of 85-120 g's (gravities) of force, while a 2-yr.-old child's neck, spinal cord, or brain stem would lethally fail if subjected to a 9-10 g's of shaking force (11-19).

'In view of these considerations, one would expect a far greater incidence of severe cervical skeletal and spinal cord injuries in infants than took place in the monkeys, and yet this type of injury has rarely if ever been documented in any SBS case to date. In view of these facts, the Shaken Baby Syndrome theory defies both reason and common observation. As a simple statement, **it is physiologically impossible**.

'As a final observation concerning "**Non-Accidental Trauma**," in which it is assumed that there is a head impact in the process of shaking, or a direct impact to the head by the caretaker, there must be substantiating evidence in the forms of head/scalp bruising and/or subgaleal (scalp) hematoma in order to justify the diagnosis of NAI. Without such evidence, the diagnosis of NAT would merely be undocumented speculation.

Reflecting these considerations, F.A. Bandak, Ph.D., a biomechanical research scientist and research professor in the Department of Neurology with the Uniformed Services University of the Health Sciences, U.S.A., and a former director of head injury research at the National Highway Traffic Safety Administration, U.S.A., wrote the following in a paper published in 2005:

> "Forceful shaking can severely injure or kill an infant. This is because the cervical spine would be severely injured and not because subdural hematomas would be caused by high head rotational accelerations. We have determined that an infant head subjected to the rotational velocity and acceleration called for in the SBS literature, **would experience forces on the infant neck far exceeding the limits for structural failure of the cervical spine.** (Emphasis mine) Furthermore, cervical spine injury from shaking can occur at much lower levels of head velocity and acceleration than those reported for the SBS (11).

(C) Bioengineers: The One and Only Scientific Discipline that Can Claim Expert Status in the Biodynamics of Whiplash Injuries, whether from Auto Accidents or from the Supposed Shaking Baby Syndrome:

Bioengineers belong to a scientific (Ph.D.) discipline that has evolved over a period of many decades as a valuable research wing of the U.S. Highway Department to study the biodynamics of whiplash injuries from auto accidents and to make safety recommendations based on these findings. However, since the biodynamics of whiplash injuries from auto accidents are identical with those involved in the violent shaking that is presumed to take place in the SBS, bioengineers have been involved in extensive investigative research in the SBS, for which Dr. Chris Van Ee has provided an extensive reference list (see below) (12). As declared below by Dr, Van Ee, it is universally accepted among members of his discipline that 1. Humans cannot generate more than a small fraction of the force required to cause brain injuries in infants by shaking alone, and 2. If such violent shaking were actually taking place, it would result in death or spinal paralysis from cervical cord injury in a large majority of infants, something that has rarely if ever been reported in the SBS literature.

(D) Chris Van Ee, Ph.D, Subject: Dynamic Biomechanical Findings on SBS-LMF

> "Scientific testing has shown that head acceleration levels from anterior/posterior human shaking of a normal 0- to 2-year-old child in the sagittal plane results in head acceleration and force levels that are much lower than those which are associated with traumatic head injury. Repeated testing of this hypothetical has shown that the head accelerations associated with shaking are far below the level associated with injury, and there is no quality data to support the SBS brain injury mechanism. Thus shaking, even if done in a fit of anger, is not expected to result in head dynamics sufficient to cause direct intracerebral trauma.

> "*Human shaking (id) may cause lethal brain stem and cervical spine injuries in a 0-to-2-year-old-child* (emphasis added), as the forces necessary for these injuries are *well below* the level needed for fatal brain injuries and are consistent with the forces that can be produced in shaking. Put another way, these neck injuries would be expected in any hypothetical-superhuman strength case of SBS where superhuman dynamics resulted in head accelerations leading to intracerebral trauma (if SBS were valid, which it is not).

> "If a 0- to 2-year-old child accidentally falls from a height of six feet and impacts head-first on a hard surface such as carpeted cement, the sudden impact has the potential to

generate sufficient head acceleration to cause fatal intrac-erebral injuries. Whether any given fall is fatal depends on a host of variables and the fall mechanics which are different in each accident, but the potential head dynamics that result from a 6-foot high fall could far exceed the tolerance associ-ated with fatal head injury.

"Intentionally impacting a 0- to 2-year-old child's head against a hard surface could easily cause fatal brain injuries that would mimic those of a fall, and today's science cannot distinguish accidental from non-accidental impacts of falls of similar magnitude, barring extraordinary signs, *e.g.* grip marks or eye-witness accounts.

"The foregoing findings are based on principles universally accepted within my field and concern scientific subject mat-ters that I am willing to testify on in this case. The findings are overwhelmingly supported by the following reference list of biomechanical tests and studies" (20).

These conclusions are further underscored by injuries of infants, properly placed in a car-seat in a high-speed head-on auto accident with severe hyperflexion whiplash of necks which caused cervical fractures, dislocations, spinal cord injury, and torn nerve roots, **but not subdural hemorrhage** (Emphasis mine)(21).

E): NonAccidental Injury (NAI)/Sudden Impact Syndrome (SIS)

There are several terms that are used interchangeably with NAI including Sudden Impact Syndrome (SIS) and abusive head trauma (AHT). All of these imply impact, primarily involving the head, which may be incidental to the assumed shaking. It could also imply a direct blow to the head or body by hand, fist, or implement.

However, for this theory to be valid it requires two elements or two pieces of diagnostic evidence. First, the child must have a significant surface head injury including prominent bruising and/ or subgaleal (scalp) hemorrhages. The former would be apparent by visual inspection. The latter would be clearly evident on head CT scans or MRIs.

Next, the diagnosis requires definitive evidence to support the "gripped" elements of shaking. For the medical expert to allege that the child was grabbed and head impacted onto a hard surface, there must be bruising imprints of gripping to provide evidence that this assumption requires. The same applies for the assumption that a child was hit severely with hand, fist, or implement. However, in a child that has had cardio-pulmonary resuscitation (CPR), soft tissue injuries must be evaluated guardedly because they may be fairly extensive in infants receiving CPR (22, 23).

Chapter 2

Subdural (Brain) Hemorrhages

(A) Suggested Differential Diagnosis of Infant Subdural Hemorrhages in Court Cases Attributed to SBS/NAI

As published in *Child Maltreatment* (2002), K.P. Hymel et al. listed 74 different conditions and diagnoses that can be caused by or associated with brain hemorrhages in infants (24). Using these reports as a basis, the following categories are suggested as starting points in recording and addressing a differential diagnosis in the medical records of SBS/NAI court cases involving brain and/or retinal hemorrhages:

Accidental Impact, Including Short Distance Falls: Plunkett (25) (2001); Reiber (26)(1993); Root (27)(1992).

Birth Trauma: As reviewed in *Nelson Textbook of Pediatrics,* 16th Edition, intracranial hemorrhage in the newborn may result from birth trauma or asphyxia. This is especially likely when the fetal head is large in proportion to the size of the mother's pelvic outlet; when for other reasons labor is prolonged; in breech or precipitate deliveries (28, 29), forceps delivery (30), or vacuum extraction(31-35). From *Spitz and Fisher's Medicolegal Investigation of Death,* 4th Edition, page 1056, the more common risk factors for infant head injuries from birth trauma include prolonged labor, abrupt labor, uncontrolled delivery of the head, macrosomia, prematurity, abnormal presentations, forceps deliveries, and vacuum extractions.

Harold Buttram M.D. and Christina England

<u>Hydrocephalus:</u> Piatt, JH (36)(1999).

<u>Prematurity and Low Birth Weights:</u> Intraventricular hemorrhages occur in 10% to 20% of very low birth weight babies (less than 1500 grams) and is thought to represent a substantial cause of morbidity and mortality in these patients (37). *Germinal Matrix and Intraventricular Hemorrhatge (GM.IVH)* is a consequence of early gestational age and the vulnerability of the immature cerebral vasculature.

<u>Hemorrhagic Disorders:</u> With findings of brain and retinal hemorrhages, hematology consultation should be routine. Late-Form Hemorrhagic Disease of the Newborn (Late-Form HDN), which is related to vitamin K deficiency, requires special attention in this category. Brain hemorrhages occur in nearly 100% of HDN cases. Spontaneous bruising is commonly prominent. The standard screening tests for hemorrhagic diseases, the prothrombin time (PT) and partial thromboplastin time (PTT), should be routinely checked with brain hemorrhages. When these are abnormally elevated, even marginally so, the PIVKA test (proteins in vitamin K absence) should be ordered, as it is specifically diagnostic for late-form HDN). Risk factors include prematurity, low birth weight, birth asphyxia, traumatic delivery, and antibiotic therapy during the perinatal period. (Antibiotics kill out beneficial intestinal flora that are essential for endogenous vitamin K production) (38). Late-form HDN is treated with vitamin K injections. Green leafy vegetables are the nutritional sources of vitamin K, which are of importance during the mother's pregnancy.

Locations of brain hemorrhages from Late-Form HDN may include virtually all areas of the brain. As an example, Demiroren K, et al. described the clinical and laboratory findings of 19 infants with intracranial hemorrhage due to vitamin K deficiency. The mean age at onset of the symptoms was 49 +/- 18 days. The localizations were parenchymal (47%), subarachnoid (47%), subdural (42%), and intraventricular (26%) (39).

(It is important to note that in my ten years reviewing records of infants with brain hemorrhages, I have seen only one instance where a PIVKA test was obtained, so that it is highly probable that many cases of Late-Form HDN are being missed by hospital physicians.)

<u>Vitamin C Deficiency (Scurvy):</u> This possibility should always be considered with subdural hemorrhages and/or unexplained bruises. Because of its unique importance, this subject will be addressed in some depth in Part III below.

<u>Spontaneous Rebleeding of Old Subdural Hematomas:</u> As described by Hymel (24), Piatt (36), and Parent (40), once subdural hemorrhages take place, they tend to take on lives of their own. As the red blood cells begin to lyse (break up) a few days following the acute hemorrhage and release their iron, microphages (scavenger cells) come in and begin taking up by phagocytosis the released iron in the form of hemosiderin. The iron is then carried out of the clot area. After a total of 3-4 weeks the iron is largely removed, at which point the hematoma enters the chronic phase and takes on the consistency of "crankcase oil," at which time it has entered the chronic phase.

About two weeks following the acute hemorrhage a thin "healing membrane" begins to form around the subdural hematoma. (As a rule, all healing of injured tissues takes place by healing membranes.) Based on electron microscopy studies, one of the characteristics of these membranes (macrocapillries) is the frequent formation of gap junctions between adjacent endothelial cells, these gaps being large enough to spill blood cells into the subdural clot area. Based on studies of Ito *et al* (41-43) it has been demonstrated that mean daily leakage of blood from the healing membranes into the subdural clot area amounted to 6.7% of their volumes, indicating continuing bleeding into the subdural cavity. These hemorrhages are partly activated by a process of fibrinolysis in the outer membranes of the subdural clots, which tends to liquefy and enlarge the clots. If the clots do slowly continue to expand, they may stretch the bridging veins traveling across the subdural space from the brain to undersurface of the skull, and once stretched beyond a certain point (some estimate 30-35%), these veins may rupture spontaneously or with minimal trauma and cause acute, sometimes massive rebleeding.

<u>Adverse Vaccine Reactions:</u> This subject is reviewed below in Section IV.

Chapter 3

Antioxidants, the Stepchildren of Modern Medicine, as Applied to SBS/NAT

Historical Perspectives

Ignatz Semmelweiss was an Austrian obstetrician who practiced his profession at a birthing center in Vienna in the mid-nineteenth century, a time when maternity death rates were an appalling 30 percent from "childbed fever," due to poor sanitary practices and conditions of the times. Semmelweiss observed that medical students would perform autopsies on the victims of childbed fever and then often go to maternity wings and deliver babies without washing their hands. Deeply troubled about the losses at the birthing center, it occurred to him that the students might be carrying some noxious substance on their hands to the mothers in the delivery wards. Acting upon this impression, he mandated that no doctor should touch a woman in labor without first washing his hands in the rather harsh soap of the times. As a result the mortality rate soon dropped from 30 percent to approximately 3 percent, while other wings in the birthing center continued with their usual 30 percent mortalities. In spite of this enormous humanitarian contribution, his work was ignored, and he became ostracized from his colleagues and remained so until his death.

Although in the field of nutrition rather than infectious disease, the story of A Kalokerinos, an Australian health officer who worked among the Australian aborigines in the 1960s and 1970s, is quite similar. When he first began his work Kalokerinos similarly became appalled by the nearly 50 percent infant mortality that was taking place. Noting signs of scurvy among some of the infants, and observing that they frequently died following immunizations, especially if ill with a viral illness, Kalokerinos began administering vitamin C supplements to the children, improving their diets, avoiding vaccines during viral illnesses (even if just a runny nose), and administering vitamin C injections during crises. Subsequently death rates dropped to three percent in his district (44).

The Australian government awarded Kalokerinos a medal of merit for his work. Also, in 1989 his work gained academic validation with the publication of a 3-volume work, *Vitamin C,* by CAB Clemetson (45). However, much after the experiences of Semmelweiss, the work of Kalokerinos has been largely overlooked or ignored by the medical profession. In my opinion this is tragic, as similar deaths among children are still taking place, although they are now in many instances being attributed to Shaken Baby Syndrome/Non-Accidental Injury (SBS/NAI).

In my 10+ years of experience with over 100 case reviews involving SBS/NAI areas, I have found record of only one case in which vitamin C blood level was tested, and even this was several weeks following hospital admission of the infant and therefore irrelevant. When the truth of this issue does become known, as it will be, I believe that vitamin C, administered orally, intramuscularly, or intravenously depending on the situation, will be found to play an indispensable protective role in the complications now being attributed to SBS/NAI.

While the recommended 30 mgs of vitamin C per day is generally adequate for a healthy infant, it may be rapidly consumed and totally inadequate when the infant is stressed or ill, as with viral or bacterial infections, or toxic chemical exposures. The common cold, for instance, has been shown to reduce vitamin C levels in the blood by 50 percent.(46) Vaccines contain numerous toxic additives and adjuvants (to be reviewed below) which create pro-inflammatory free radicals. All vaccine adjuvants are pro-oxidants that drain the body's supply of antioxidants including vitamin C (47). Another risk factor may be the use of microwave ovens for heating infant formulas. Also, fruits and vegetables need to be reasonably fresh, as vitamin C content declines with aging.

(**NOTE**: In an article entitled "A role for IFN- Alpha Beta in virus infection-induced sensitization to endotoxin, (LA Doughty *et al, Journal of Immunology* 2001)(48), the authors confirmed the importance of avoiding vaccines during viral illnesses, as originally observed and recommended by Kalokerinos, in their findings that "underlying viral infections can heighten sensitivity and worsen worsen cytokine-mediated disease following secondary inflammatory challenges," (which would include vaccines and their pro-inflammatory adjuvants.)

Elevated Blood Histamine as Cause of Capillary Fragility and Bleeding from Scurvy

Far from being uncommon, vitamin C deficiency still does occur in the Western World. When people attending a Health Maintenance Organization (HMO) clinic in Tempe, Arizona, were tested for plasma vitamin C, it was found to be depleted (between 0.2 and 0.5 mgs/100 ml) in 30 percent of subjects, and to be deficient (below 0.2 mgs/100 ml) in 6 percent (49).

As reviewed by Clemetson, when the human plasma ascorbic acid level falls below 0.2 mg/ml, the whole blood histamine level is doubled or quadrupled. (50) Blood histamine is also increased by vaccines or toxoids, by stresses such as heat or cold, and by various drugs in guinea pigs (51). Vitamin C has been shown to inactivate tetanus toxin (52 and diphtheria toxin (53). It has been shown that *bleeding from scurvy results from increased blood histamine, or histaminemia, which causes separation of endothelial cells from one another in capillaries and small venules* (54). This process may result in subperiosteal hemorrhages, the latter resulting in callus-like bone swellings commonly misinterpreted as fractures, extensive spontaneous bruising, and subdural hemorrhages which were included in early descriptions of classical scurvy (55-56).

The Human Infant Brain: Uniquely Susceptible to Lipid Peroxidation

Although an infant's brain receives 15 percent of normal cardiac output, it utilizes nearly 25 percent of the body's oxygenation (57). In addition to being a highly oxygenated organ, the vulnerability of the human brain to harmful peroxidation rests on the fact that it has by far the highest fat content of any organ of the body with membrane lipids constituting 60 percent of the solid matter (58). In addition, both brain and retina contain a relatively high percentage of the omega-3 polyunsaturated fatty acid, docosahexaenoic acid (DHA)(59-65) which serves as a primary building block of the membranes of these structures. The DHA and other polyunsaturated fatty acids are high in energetics, but they are far more unstable and prone to pro-inflammatory peroxidation (rancidity) than saturated fats (59-65).

By way of explanation, the term "lipid peroxidation" refers to free-radical generation from a series of chain reactions, which can be very damaging if the process is prolonged. "Free-radicals" in turn refer to atoms with unpaired electrons, which results in heightened instability and reactivity. The end result of abnormally prolonged lipid peroxidation may be abnormal brain inflammation and brain swelling.

In essence, the brain might be compared with highly inflammable dry grass or brush enclosed with elevated oxygen levels, needing only a spark to set off a conflagration of inflammatory lipid peroxidation. In all likelihood, vaccine adjuvants provide this spark far more often than generally realized.

In addition, the infant's immature brain and nervous system tissues are going through an extended period of rapid growth and development, which also bring heightened vulnerability to cellular damage. As reported by R.I. Haynes *et al* (66)(2005)(*Journal of Comparative Neurology*), cerebral axons (lengthy extensions of brain cells) achieve approximately one-fourth of adult level from the 24th to the 34th weeks during pregnancy, with rapid axonal growth and elongation taking place between 21 weeks during

16

pregnancy and 24 weeks following birth. Onset of myelin development (fatty coating that protects nerve cells and provides nerve
impulse insulation), does not commence until 14 weeks following
birth with gradual progression to adult-like staining at 32 to 52
weeks. *It is during this period of furious brain growth, limited myelin
protection, and increased vulnerabilities that infants receive over 21
vaccines, according to today's recommended schedule.*

Hazards of Free Iron In and Around the Brain

Standard pediatric texts list prolonged labor, fetal malpresentation,
and large babies as risk factors for significant brain hemorrhages.
Tauscher *et al* reported an association between histologic chorioamnionitis (inflammation of the placenta) and brain hemorrhage
in preterm infants (67). Intracerebral hemorrhage occurs in up
to 50 percent of very low-birth-weight infants and is thought to
represent a substantial cause of morbidity and mortality in these
infants (68). Small subdural hemorrhages (SDH) are not uncommon
in uncomplicated births and asymptomatic term newborns. Based
on magnetic resonance imaging (MRI), Whitby *et a l*(69)(2004)
reported subdurals in 9 of 111 infants in 2004, all of which had
resolved favorably when MRIs were repeated one month later. V.J.
Rooks *et al* (70)(2008) performed MRI scans on 101 term infants
at 72 hours, 2 weeks, one month, and 3 months. *Forty-six had
asymptomatic SDH within 72 hours of delivery.* All 46 had supraten-
torial SDH in the posterior cranium. Forty three percent also had
infratentorial SDH. Most SDH were < 3 mm in sizes, all of which
were resolved within one month. Larger hematomas dissolved
within 3 months.

Consequently, small hemorrhages are not uncommon even in uncomplicated childbirths, but little consideration has been given to
the residual iron. As the red blood cells begin to lyse (break up) and
release their iron following a hemorrhage, a process that takes place
in two or three weeks, the iron is scavenged by white blood cells
and carried into nearby tissues in the form of hemosiderin (71).

Free-iron in and around the brain also may result when there are
critical drops in levels of vitamin C following administration of

vaccines, followed in turn by a precipitous rise in serum histamine bringing increased capillary fragility and leakage of blood into and around the brain.

It is known that iron overload in the liver, pancreas, and kidneys can be very destructive, a condition known has hemochromatosis. The concern here is that residual iron in and around the brain from an earlier brain hemorrhages, such as from birth trauma, may act as a lighted fuse that could ignite a firestorm of lipid peroxidation in the brain following vaccines (72).

Chapter 4

Increased Hazards of Vaccines in Preterm Infants

In a report in by Sen *et al* in *Acta Paediatr* (73)(2001), case histories of 45 preterm babies who were vaccinated with DPT/Hib (diphtheria, tetanus toxoids, pertussis, and Haemophilus influenzae type B conjugate) in the neonatal intensive care unit of the Royal Gwent Hospital, Newport, UK between January 1993 and December 1998 were studied retrospectively. Apparent adverse events were noted in 17 of 45 (37.8 %) babies, 9 (20%) of whom had major events , i.e. apnea, bradycardia, or desaturations. Age at 70 days or less was significantly associated with increased risk.

After observing the occurrence of apnea, usually associated with bradycardia, in two preterm infants following immunization with DTP and HIB, Sanchez *et al* (74)(*Journal of Pediatrics,*1997) conducted a prospective surveillance of 97 (50 girls and 47 boys) preterm infants younger than 37 weeks gestation who were immunized with DTP (94 also received Haemophilus b at the same time) in the neonatal intensive care unit in Texas, USA to assess the frequency of adverse reactions, and in particular the occurrence of apnea. For each infant data were recorded for a 3-day period before and after receipt of the immunizations. Their studies showed that apnea occurred in 34 infants (34 %) after immunizations, and 11 (11%) had at least 50 % increase in the number of apneic and bradycardia episoces in the 72 hours after immunization. This occurred primarily among smaller preterm infants who were immunized at a lower weight and had experienced more severe apnea of prematurity.

Slack *et al* (1994)(75) from the United Kingdom reported that four premature infants developed apneas severe enough to warrant resuscitation after immunization with diphtheria, pertussis, and tetanus (DPT) and Haemophilus influenza type b. One required intubation and ventilation.

A study on primary immunization of 239 premature infants with gestational ages of less than 35 weeks by M Pourcyrous *et al.* (76) (*Journal of Pediatrics,* 2007), was conducted to determine the incidence of cardio-respiratory events and abnormal C-reactive protein (CRP) elevations associated with administration of a single vaccine or multiple vaccines simultaneously at or about two months age. (CRP is a standard blood test indicator for body inflammation, which in the present study would represent brain inflammation.) CRP levels and cardio-respiratory manifestations were monitored for three days following immunizations in a neonatal intensive care unit sponsored by the University of Tennessee. Elevations of CRP levels occurred in 70% of infants administered single vaccines and in 85% of those given multiple vaccines, 43% of which reached abnormal levels. Overall, 16% of infants had vaccine-associated cardiorespiratory events with episodes of apnea (cessation of breathing) and bradycardia (slowing of pulse). **It can be reasonably assumed that the cardiorespiratory events and CRP elevations primarily reflect brain inflammation and swelling following the vaccines. Most important for our present topic, intraventricular (brain) hemorrhages occurred in 17% of infants receiving single vaccines, with 24% incidence in those receiving multiple vaccines. For the first time this study documents that a significant incidence of brain hemorrhages can result from vaccines in vulnerable infants.** (Personal emphasis)

The special importance of the Pourcyrous study was in being the first to assess the role of brain inflammation in adverse vaccine reactions In so doing it has provided a unified theory of adverse vaccine reactions:

- Brain Inflammation, as indicated by C-Reactive Proteins.

- Brain swelling, which always takes place with in-flammation as one of its cardinal signs.
- Potentially lethal cardio-respiratory events.
- Brain hemorrhages.

The Pourcyrous study also raises a question. Why were the brain hemorrhages in the study intraventricular rather than subdural, the latter now being associated with the Shaken Baby Syndrome? The answer is that the Pourcyrous study was performed on preterm infants, some born less than 30 weeks term, in whom intraventricular hemorrhages are known to be characteristic. This may be due to the infant brain/skull interactions at these different stages of development. In preterm infants the skull would be highly flaccid, providing little if any resistance to a swollen (edematous) brain.

In term infants, in contrast, the inner surface of the skull presents a relatively firm surface, and when brain inflammation and edema take place from vaccines (77-79), it would require very little brain swelling for the outer surface of the brain to impact against the inner surface of the skull and, tourniquet-like, to cut off the passive outflow of blood from the subdural venous network. With cranial arterial blood coming in at much higher pressures, this would pre-dictably cause a precipitous rise in intracerebral venous pressure, the true cause of many subdural hematomas.

According to a report by W Squier and J Mack (80)(2009), most childhood subdural hemorrhages are identified in infants 0-4 months of age, a time when the subdural compartment consists of 10-15 layers of loosely arranged flake-like cells with fluid between them and few intercellular junctions (81). *Because of the looseness of the dural fiber layers at this age, it would be highly permeable.* Under these circumstances it is predictable that a rapid surge in intracerebral venous pressure would rapidly force blood from the subdural venous network into these loosely connected and highly permeable subdural membranes, the true cause of many subdural hemorrhages now being attributed to SBS/NAT. The same tourniquet-like process would also cause retinal hemorrhages.

Chapter 5

Pro-inflammatory Vaccine Adjuvants: Aluminum & Peanut Oil

In what may be the most comprehensive review to date on the pathophysiology of adverse vaccine reactions, Russell Blaylock has compiled a mass of evidence that repeated stimulation of the brain's immune system results in intense reactions of microglial and astraglia cells, which serve as the brain's immune system, with each successive series of vaccinations. This is primarily the result **vaccine adjuvants** that are added expressly for that purpose (82-84).

In explanation, microglia and astrocytes are first-line-immunological responder cells located in the brain that defend against foreign infectious invaders. Normally this response, such as to a viral infection, is of limited duration and harmless to the brain. However, when microglia and astrocytes are over-stimulated for prolonged periods, which vaccine adjuvants are designed to bring about, this extended activation can be very destructive to the brain.

Because of the critical dependence of the developing brain on a timed sequence of cytokine and excitatory amino acid fluctuations, according to Blaylock, sequential vaccinations can result in alterations of this critical process that will not only result in synaptic and dendritic loss, but abnormal (nerve) pathway development. *When microglia are excessively activated by vaccines, especially chronically, they secrete a number of **proinflammatory** cytokines, free radicals, lipid peroxidation products, and the two excitotoxins, glutamate and quinolenic acid, which may become proinflammatory and highly* *destructive when activated for prolonged periods.* (Emphasis added) This process was suggested as the principle mechanisms resulting in the pathological as well as clinical features of autism (82).

Vaccine adjuvants are substances added to vaccine formulations during manufacturing that are designed to boost and prolong the overall immune system response when the vaccine is injected. For many years two forms of aluminum, (*aluminum hydroxide and aluminum phosphate*) were the only compounds specifically authorized by the FDA to be used as vaccine adjuvants, although other additives may also have pro-inflammatory effects, prominent among which isThimerosal (50 percent ethyl mercury), which is still added to a number of vaccines as a preservative (85). In addition, mercury is commonly used in the manufacturing process of vaccines, which leaves "traces" as residues. Even these trace amounts are potentially toxic because of the universally recognized principle of toxicology that combinations of toxins will increase toxicity exponentially; that is, two toxins will increase toxicity 10-fold, or three toxins increase toxicity 100-fold. In vaccines special attention should be given to the two toxic heavy metals, aluminum and mercury, each noted for its potential toxicity.The same principle applies in other classes of toxic chemicals 1-4). In view of these findings, Russel Blaylock has referred to the inconsolable, high-pitched cry that commonly occurs following infant vaccinations as an "encephalitic cry."

Unlabeled Peanut Oil

In a newly released book, *The History of the Peanut Allergy Epidemic* (86), Heather Fraser thoroughly documents how highly allergenic peanut oil came to be used in vaccinations without being listed on the package insert. With her background as a historian and mother of a child with a fatal peanut allergy, Ms Fraser wrote from personal knowledge and experience.

By definition, a vaccine adjuvant is a substance that is added to enhance and prolong antibody responses to viral and bacterial vaccines, thereby enhancing their effectiveness. Aluminum has been in use for this purpose since the earliest days of vaccine programs. As outlined by Heather Fraser, the first use of peanut oil came about in 1945 in Alexander Fleming's newly discovered penicillin. The original problem with penicillin was that a single dose of would last only three hours before being excreted by the kidneys.

This problem was solved by an Army Medical Corps Captain, Monroe Romansky, who had discovered a method of prolonging the action of penicillin by mixing it with 4 % to 4.8% beeswax and peanut oil. This was a simple solution to the problem. As the body metabolized the oil, the drug was released slowly into the system (87). In 1948 doctors began to use PAM (penicillin with aluminum monostearate), an aqueous solution suspended in peanut oil, which produced desirable penicillin blood levels for 24 to 26 hours.

The first use of peanut oil in vaccines was reported in 1964 by the *New York Times,* which announced that pharmaceutical giant Merck had begun to use a new vaccine ingredient that promised to extend immunity against influenza, polio, and other illnesses (88). It was called Adjuvant 65-4, as it contained up to 65% peanut oil as well as Arlacel A, aluminum stearate and other ingredients. As in penicillin, the peanut oil surrounds the vaccine antigens. When injected into the muscle, the oil was gradually metabolized by the body providing a sustained release of the other ingredients and *producing 13-fold higher levels of antibodies than had formerly taken place from aqueous vaccine formulations* (89). (Emphasis added)

In the 1970s and 1980s, following modifications of the original adjuvant 65-4, the use of peanut oil in vaccines became common practice (90-92).

As tabulated by Heather Fraser, it was during this time period that the incidence of peanut allergies began to rise in exponential proportions, as well as increases in Guillain-Barre Syndrome (93). which began in 1976 following vaccination with a hastily prepared flu vaccine. Over 4,000 complaints of damage from this vaccine were settled by the US government for $72 million. A flood of vaccine-related lawsuits involving DPT escalated from one suit in 1979 to 255 in 1986.

However, this litigious environment was changed by the National

Childhood Vaccine Injury Act of 1986 and its compensating program in 1988, which forced parents to exhaust the "no fault" government alternative before being allowed to sue vaccine makers directly. This easing on vaccine makers made way for the dramatic intensification in the pediatric vaccine schedules and for vaccination programs targeting preschoolers.

During the period of expanding pediatric vaccination in western countries, the prevalence of peanut and other food allergies accelerated. Unseen by the public, hospital emergency room records in Australia, the UK, and the USA documented the upward momentum of food anaphylaxis admissions of children under five. In the USA, ER records showed an increase in anaphylaxis discharges between 1992 and 1994 from 467 per 100,000 to 671. The number jumped to 876 in 1995 (94). A 1991 USA study determined that 90 percent of all food allergy fatalities were due to ingestion of peanut/tree nuts (95).

Revisiting Antioxidants

As final pieces of evidence connecting the pro-inflammatory effects of vaccine adjuvants/additives with antioxidant deficiencies, as the true cause of many subdural brain hemorrhages now being attributed to inflicted child abuse, in a cross-sectional analysis of the third National Health and Nutrition Examination Survey data, Ford *et al*(96) reported that C-Reactive Protein concentrations were inversely and significantly associated with concentrations of retinaol, retinyl esters, vitamin C, alpha carotene, beta carotene, lycopene, cryptoxanthin, lutein or zeaxanthin, and selenium C after adjustment for age, gender, race-ethnicity, education, body mass index (BMI), leisure-time physical activity, and aspirin use. Furthermore, Wannamethee *et al* (97) reported a significant inverse association of dietary and plasma vitamin C and fruit and vegetable intakes with biomarkers of inflammation in a cross-sectional study of 3258 men aged 60-69 years who had no history of cardiovascular disease or diabetes. Wannamethee *et al* concluded that vitamin C has anti-inflammatory effects and is associated with an attenuation of endothelial dysfunction.

Chapter 6

Vaccine Combinations and Immune Paralysis

Basis of the Human Immune System Prior to Introduction of Vaccines

The human newborn comes into the world with residual antibodies from the maternal blood stream which, in the absence of breast feeding, provide immunologic protection for about six months, for measles up to 12 months. Otherwise the newborn immune system is largely rudimentary, *requiring a series of microbe challenges to become fully functional,* a process requiring two or three years. Without these challenges the immune system would remain weak and vestigial.

The immune system is divided into two major classes: *Cellular immunity,* located in the mucous membranes of the respiratory and gastrointestinal tracts and their respective lymph nodes, and *humoral immunity,* with production of antigen-specific antibodies by plasma cells in the bone marrow. For eons of time the mucous membranes of the respiratory and gastrointestinal tracts have been the primary sites of microbe entry into the body so that, of necessity, cellular immunity has evolved as the primary immune defense system of the body, with humoral immunity playing a secondary or back up role.

Both classes are governed by TH lymphocytes, the "T" referring to the thymus gland from which they are derived and the "H" referring to helper activity. Early in life these uncommitted or "naïve" TH lymphocytes are differentiated into either armed Th1 cells, which govern in cellular immunity, or Th2 cells, which govern in humoral immunity. It has been found that this differentiation has been profoundly affected by cytokines, which are produced by lymphocytes and which serve as chemical messengers. The two cytokines, interleukin 12 and interferon gamma promote and govern Th1 cells, while interleukins 4, 5, 6, and 10 promote and govern Th2 cells (98). Once one subset becomes dominant, it is difficult to shift the response to the other subset, as the cytokines from one tend to dominate the other.

Why are these technicalities important? Current vaccine programs are in effect attempting to groom the humoral system into the *primary immune system* of the body, a role it can never fully or effectively play. *The cellular immune system, in contrast, lacking former challenges of the so-called "minor childhood diseases" of former times (measles, mumps, chicken pox, and rubella) may be going through the process of atrophy of disuse,* also being further compromised by the immunosuppressant effects of combination-viral-vaccines. It is true there are many other forms of viral challenges today, but only these four significantly challenged and therefore strengthened the immunity of the epithelial and endothelial tissues of the body and their associated organs.

Furthermore, current childhood vaccine programs may in a sense be turning childhood immune systems "inside-out," with the humoral system being thrown into an abnormal dominance over the cellular system. This in turn results in the suppression of the cytokine, interleukin 12, on which the cellular system is largely dependant. (106, 107)

The MMR (Measles-Mumps-Rubella) Vaccine

The name of Dr. Andrew Wakefield will probably be familiar to most people reading these lines in connection with his original description of the "autistic-colitis syndrome" and his work in tracing back the cause to intestinal implantations of the measles virus following the MMR (Measles-Mumps-Rubella) vaccines. Although controversial now, it is predicted that Wakefield's work in this area will in time come to be recognized as a major advancement in the history of medicine (99-101). As Wakefield correctly pointed out, the measles, mumps, and rubella vaccines had been administered separately since the 1940s with only slight rise in the incidence of autism, but with an abrupt spiking in incidence following introduction of the MMR vaccine in the USA in 1978 (102-103).

Early in their investigations Wakefield *et al* astutely checked back into the records of public health departments in the United Kingdom and found reports of autism occurring among children contracting two of these diseases simultaneously, such as chicken pox and measles or rubella and measles.

In addition to the Blaylock model of microglial overstimulation (82), there are two plausible explanations for increases in autism following the MMR vaccine: First, protein sequences in the measles virus have been found to have a similarities to those in brain tissues (104), so that by process of mimicry, the formation of antibodies against the measles virus would tend to cross react adversely with brain tissues. Second, and probably far more important, a healthy immune system requires both a vigorous humoral (antibody production) system and vigorous cellular immune system, the latter being governed by the thymus gland. Viruses are inherently immunosuppressant in contrast to bacterial infections which stimulate the immune system, as reflected in the fact that viral infections generally lower white blood counts. *The measles virus is exceptionally potent in this regard*, *being powerfully suppressive to cellular immunity* (105-107). Consequently the combining of three viral vaccines into a single combination may substantially increase the immunosuppressive viral effect bringing about in varying degrees an immune paralysis of the cellular immune system in recipients. In support of this, Wakefield *et al* have demonstrated the measles virus in intestinal lymph nodes of children with the autistic-colitis syndrome, in which the only exposures to the measles virus were from the MMR vaccine (101).

A Case Report: Dramatic Anaphylactic (Anamnestic) Response to Vaccines that May Have Contained Unlabeled Peanut Oil.

A case is presented of an infant born at 29 and 5/7 weeks gestation with very low birth weight of 1,600 grams (3.52 lbs) and a prominent left facial hemagioma. Following routine 4-month vaccines, the mother observed significant though transient puffiness of the hemangioma. A head CT scan ordered on the 6-month visit showed frontal lobe atrophy and mildly dilated ventricles but no acute hemorrhage. By pure coincidence, routine 6-month vaccines were administered later the same morning as the head CT scan, followed within moments by loud, high-pitched crying and spurting of blood "all over" from the facial hemangioma. A brain MRI two days later showed extensive bilateral subdural hematomas. Although these were attributed to "non-accidental trauma" by hospital physicians, the dramatic reactions from the 6-month vaccines, including the subdural hematomas, almost certainly represented an anamnestic allergic response from the 4-month vaccines in which the aluminum adjuvant and the unlabeled peanut oil adjuvant would have played prominent roles.

Adverse Effects of Early Cord Clamping (119):

Before birth, the placenta breathes for the child, feeds it, and excretes for it. After birth, the child's lungs, gut, and kidneys must take over these functions that are controlled by the child's brain. During birth, blood is transferred from the placenta to the child so that the lungs, gut, kidneys, <u>and brain</u> can function well. Immediate cord clamping following birth (ICC) keeps a significant portion of blood in the placenta and averts the forceful surge this blood would bring which is essential for opening up formerly dormant vascular networks to the lungs, gut, kidneys, and especially the brain, the latter being the most vulnerable of all body organs to any degree of hypoxia following birth.

According to Erasmus Darwin, 1770:

> "Another thing very injurious to the child is the tying and cutting of the navel string too soon; which should always be

left till the child has not only repeatedly breathed but till all pulsation in the cord ceases. As otherwise the child is much weaker than it ought to be, a portion of the blood being left in the placenta, which ought to have been in the child."

The Brilliant Work of Dr. Mohammed Ali Al-Bayati in SBS Cases

In an analytical scheme so simple that a child could understand, and yet so brilliant that no one else has thought of it (to the best of my knowledge), Dr. M.A. Al-Bayati has has evaluated the growth rates from standard developmental graphs of infant weights, lengths, and head circumferences before and after vaccines, showing that vaccine can reduce skeletal and head circumference growth in a time-related fashion. (120) However, the head circumference can also increase within hours following vaccines due to vaccine-induced brain inflammation with secondary edema (121, 122). Subdural hemorrhages from vaccines can also cause time-related increases in head circumferences, which places heavy responsibility on pediatricians to perform regular head circumference measurements during routine childhood visits.

Conclusions

The human infant brain has heightened vulnerability to inflammation due to its relatively high oxygen levels and high fat content, a large portion of which consists of polyunsaturated fatty acids, which are high in energetics but relatively unstable and susceptible to damaging peroxidation.

The Pourcyrous study may prove to be a pivotal landmark in the history of medicine. The first study of its kind, it provides a unified theory of adverse vaccine reactions with documented brain inflammation, as indicated by increases levels of C-Reactive proteins in 70 percent of infants administered a single vaccine and 85 percent of those administered multiple vaccines. Brain swelling (edema) would automatically follow as one of the cardinal signs of inflammation; brain swelling in turn would immediately impact against the inner surface of the skull, cutting off (tourniquet-like) the passively outflow of blood through the subdural venous network. With arterial intracranial blood coming in at much higher pressures, this in turn would cause a precipitous rise in intracranial venous pressure. As the final connecting point, the subdural membrane in early infancy consists of 10-15 loosely connected flake-like cells separated by fluid, rendering them highly permeable and vulnerable to the precipitous rise in venous pressure, the true cause of subdural hemorrhages in many of these cases, in my opinion.

Before publication of the Pourcyrous study, vaccine issues could rarely be presented successfully in court in SBS/NAI cases. Since its publication, the potential role of vaccines in these cases cannot be legitimately denied.

Studies by Ommaya (5)(1968), Duhaime (12)(1987), Prange (15) (2003), Bandak, (17)(2005), and many others have demonstrated that, if the presumed violent shaking were actually taking place in SBS cases, it would result in a large majority of fatalities or cervical spinal cord injuries (paraplegia) from upper cervical spinal cord and brain stem damage. This is because by far the greatest force from the shaking would be concentrated at the junction between upper cervical spine and the lower surface of the skull, where the brain stem is located.

Observations of more than 10 years in these cases has revealed a general pattern of precipitous diagnoses of inflicted child abuse by hospital physicians without adequate medical workups to rule out other common potential causes of the findings. These include head injuries or fractures from birth trauma; hydrocephalus; hemorrhagic disorders, among which late-form hemorrhagic disease of the newborn (HDN) from vitamin K deficiency; antioxidant deficiencies, especially vitamin C, as a contributory cause of brain hemorrhages and/or bruising; and metabolic fractures, among which rickets is known to be common. In personal experiences of over ten years in these cases I have seen only one case in which the PIVKA test (proteins in vitamin K absence) was performed, although there were many cases with prolonged bleeding studies in which the PIVKA should have been performed. Plasma ascorbate should be mandatory in any case with brain hemorrhages and/

or bruises. Blood tests for 25-hydroxy vitamin D, parathormone, calcium, phosphorus, alkaline phosphatase should also be mandatory in any infant with unexplained fractures, as well as a dietary history of the mother during the pregnancy. I have yet to see a case of infant fractures in which a maternal dietary history was investigated in the medical records.

Regarding 5 in 1 vaccines, each individual vaccine in these combinations has a tainted history, with many hundreds of thousands of reactions having been reported world wide. These reactions include encephalitis, convulsions (sometimes leading to epilepsy), uncontrollable screaming, exceptionally high temperatures, severe brain damage, Guillain-Barre Syndrome, and death. The common denominators linking all these vaccines are various chemicals and toxins, including thimerosal (50 percent mercury), aluminium, and formaldehyde, all of which are known to be neurotoxic. Mercury and aluminum are both linked to Alzheimer's disease.

Many babies born prematurely are very sick babies. They can have a variety of problems including infections and respiratory problems. An irreconcilable contradiction in these situations is that, while preterm infants are targeted for vaccinations to protect them because they are seen as high risk, they are far more vulnerable to the numerous toxic adjuvants and additives in vaccines. Vaccines are dated from day of birth with no allowances for risks of prematurity, as demonstrated by the frequency of intraventricular hemorrhages in the Pourcyrous study, with 17 percent hemorrhages in infants administered one vaccine, and 24 percent in infants administered multiple vaccines.

It is very clear that the greater the number of vaccines administered to preterm infants, the greater will be the numbers of parents and caretakers that are falsely accused of SBS/NAI (118).

Part 2:

Five in One Vaccines

by Christina England

Chapter 7

A Dangerous Combination

The five-in-one vaccine is a pentavalent combination vaccine, combining a total of five separate vaccines into one vial. This vaccine is usually given to a baby in three doses, two months, four months, six months. The vaccine although given in one syringe, is an amalgamation of the diphtheria, tetanus, pertussis (whooping cough), Haemophilus influenzae type b (the main cause of childhood meningitis and pneumonia), and polio vaccines—or DTaP, Hib B, IPV or DTaP, Hib B, and dropping the polio and opting for hep B, which is for hepatitis B.

Taking the history of each vaccine in turn, we can quickly establish that each of these vaccines has a tainted history, with many adverse reactions. Is it a wise move to put all these highly toxic and potentially dangerous vaccines into one syringe? Surely as a result, we should not be surprised to see the adverse reactions soar. Only time will tell, but how many precious lives will be lost and how many more parents will be falsely accused of shaken baby syndrome (SBS) as the world embarks on yet another "government vaccine experiment"?

Diphtheria, Tetanus, Pertussis or DTP/DTaP

Let us first examine closely the DTP, which later changed to the DTaP and will be discussed later. The DTP was a vaccine first introduced to the vaccine schedules during the 1930s and has been problematic from the onset, when adverse reactions quickly began to emerge. In 1948, Randolph Byers and Frederick Moll, both of the

Harvard Medical School and the Federal Drug Administration, became so concerned that they carried out tests and soon concluded that the DTP could produce severe neurological problems in some children. Their tests and conclusions were later published in the medical journal *Pediatrics*.

Professor Gordon T. Stewart first began to have serious concerns about the adverse reactions to vaccines in the 1940s to 1950s. One of his earliest papers on vaccines was written in 1951 and entitled "Infectivity and virulence of tubercle bacilli." Lancet 2; 562[123]. In the early 1970s, he began to write a series of papers raising serious concerns that he had in reference to the pertussis vaccine (whooping cough), one of the components of the DTP.

Stewart[124] wrote that from a group of 1127 children in whom signs of brain damage were reported after injections of vaccines containing the pertussis antigen, the first 197 cases with good documentation of adverse events were chosen for further study. He wrote:

> In these children, 291 reactions had been reported, usually of screaming attacks (68), convulsions (87), collapse (17), or one or more of these signs (99), within twenty-four hours of injection.

> The 197 children received a total of 435 injections of the DTP (one injection only, 54; two injections, 57; three, 77; four, 9) A total of 121 children reacted to one injection, 47 to two, 25 to three, and 4 to four injections. Of the 123 who reacted badly to the first injection, 63 received one or more subsequent injections, to which all but 3 reacted again similarly or more severely. Reactions reported were mainly described as uncontrollable screaming or convulsions, which usually occurred within twenty-four hours of receiving the vaccine. In most cases, these reactions were reported to GP's, health visitors, or clinics during or soon after the incidents; but in 52 children in whom the reaction subsided, reports were not made until the next injection was due. Many children were taken to the hospital as emergencies; others were referred to pediatricians

or pediatric neurologists later, when it was apparent that the child was not recovering.

At around the time that Professor Stewart was writing papers on his concerns, unease was arising in many quarters. In 1978 after fighting for many years with the UK government for a compensation scheme, Rosemary Fox, of the Association of Parents of Vaccine Damaged Children, an organization she set up because her own daughter suffered brain damage after the vaccine, took her complaints and concerns about the DTP vaccine to the European Court of Human Rights. Her complaint[125] began:

> *On behalf of the Association of Parents of Vaccine Damaged Children, I have collected details of 287 (to date) cases of healthy children who, as a result of vaccination, suffered death almost immediately – 6 cases death later followed prolonged illness – 4 cases last year, or brain damage to such an extent that their lives have been completely destroyed and in many cases are at risk.*
>
> *In no case was the possibility of such a risk discussed beforehand with parents, or was there any public knowledge of risk. In all cases, parents accepted vaccination in the belief that this was for the protection of their healthy child.*

Not a lot has changed over the years, as the complaint stated:

1. *The British Government acknowledges that no immunizing procedure is entirely free from risk or from adverse reactions. In the Therapeutic Substances Act, 1956, by the British Parliament, vaccines are described as* **"substances the purity or potency of which cannot be adequately tested by chemical means."**

2. *The protection of the individual vaccinee is not now the sole purpose of routine vaccination programs;* **vaccination is concerned with maintaining or promoting national immunity.**

3. *Although no vaccination is legally compulsory in the United Kingdom, the immunization scheme is not truly based on voluntary acceptance or fully informed consent. A high*

> *acceptance rate is maintained because all parents are strongly*
> *encouraged to accept "protection for their child." They are*
> *never informed that vaccination is not solely for individual*
> *protection or **that for some children vaccination can mean***
> ***death or serious injury.***

Her complaint highlights the fact that governments are aware that vaccines can cause serious injury but are willing to "sacrifice a few" in an attempt to protect what they call "herd immunity."

Fox was successful in winning her battle and won each vaccine damaged child a sum of £10,000.

Complaints and problems surrounding the DTP continued to come in from around the world. Harris L. Coulter[126] said that there was much concern regarding the DTP, which in his opinion was by then seen to be responsible for the growing numbers of sudden infant death or SIDS. He wrote:

> *Matters came to a crisis when William C. Torch, M.D., Director*
> *of Child Neurology, Department of Pediatrics, University of*
> *Nevada School of Medicine, at the 34th Annual Meeting of the*
> *American Academy of Pediatrics, presented a study linking*
> *the DPT shot with SIDS. Torch concluded: "These data show*
> *that DPT vaccination may be a generally unrecognized major*
> *cause of sudden infant and early childhood death, and that the*
> *risks of immunization may outweigh its potential benefits. A*
> *need for re-evaluation and possible modification of current*
> *vaccination procedures is indicated by this study.*

Coulter also wrote about another study around the same time showing that other professionals also had became concerned Larry J. Baraff, Wendy J. Ablon, and Robert C. Weiss.[127]

> *Another article on the SIDS-vaccination relationship, fortu-*
> *nately of far superior quality, is Larry J. Baraff, Wendy J. Ablon,*
> *and Robert C. Weiss, "Possible Temporal Association Between*
> *Diphtheria-Tetanus Toxoid-Pertussis Vaccination and Sudden*
> *Infant Death Syndrome." (Pediatric Infectious Diseases 2:1*

[January, 1983], 7-11). The authors adopted a simpler, in-tuitively obvious method of investigation and concluded that there is, indeed, a "temporal association" between the DPT shot and sudden infant death. They found that 382 cases of SIDS were recorded in Los Angeles County between January 1, 1979, and August 23, 1980, and they simply interviewed the parents of 145 of these cases, either in person or by telephone. They asked: 1) the baby's sex, 2) the age at death, 3) the last visit to a physician or nurse prior to death, 4) the date of the last vaccination, 5) the name and telephone number of the physician or nurse, and 6) the type of immunization given.

They found a statistically significant excess of deaths in the first day and the first week after vaccination, i.e., a "temporal association." They rejected the use of a "control group," and instead relied on the intuitively obvious assumption that "there should be no temporal association between DPT immunization and SIDS were there no causal relationship between these two events." I have not found any criticism of this article for relying on "anecdotal evidence." This study was not financed by the US Government but apparently by the UCLA School of Medicine and the Los Angeles County Department of Health Services.

It is possible that a percentage of these children had, in fact, suffered from bleeds to the brain; but at that time, without the availability of the technology in use today, it was difficult to say what was causing these infants distress or indeed their premature deaths. The first scanners able to detect this sort of brain injury did not come into use until the mid seventies, as the first CAT or CT scanner (CT scanning combines special x-ray equipment with sophisticated computers to produce multiple images or pictures of the inside of the body)was not invented by Godfrey Hounsfield until 1971. Before the invention of the CT scanner, it was not possible to produce detailed pictures of patients' brains; however, with this machine, doctors were first able to show the medical usefulness of scanning. The CT scanner was the first type of scanner to be adopted in substantial numbers for medicine and set the pattern for other scanning technologies. Without this technology available to them, the neurologists examining possible vaccine damaged infants had little way of knowing for certain whether these children were displaying symptoms that medical professionals these days attribute to SBS.

Due to the growing number of side effects being recognized, in 1991, the new DTaP vaccine was licensed in the United States. The pertussis component of this vaccine is a more purified, "acellular" version, which was said to produce fewer side effects than the original vaccine, which by now had been identified as having a high rate of side effects, including brain injury and death. DTaP, which is also sometimes called DTPa or TDaP, is a combined vaccine against diphtheria, tetanus, and pertussis, in which the pertussis component is acellular. The acellular vaccine uses selected antigens of the pertussis pathogen to induce immunity; because it uses fewer antigens than the whole cell vaccines, it is considered safer, but it is also more expensive. Most of the developed world has now switched to the DTaP, but developing countries still continue to use the DTP.

The acellular vaccine was considered by many professionals to be safer, showing what was believed to be substantially fewer side effects. However, more recent evidence has contraindicated this, showing that there has been little change to the figures of serious adverse reactions being reported.

Kris Gaublomme[128] wrote in his paper "Acellular Pertussis—The International Vaccination," that data on the safety issues of the acellular vaccine were contradictory.

> *The Japanese study (I) e.g. mentions that "the vaccine does not have detectable side-effects", whereas the introduction of the same article says that "it is less than one-tenth as toxic as whole-cell vaccine ... ". How can a quantitative comparison be made if there is "no detectable side-effect" at all? Poland (8) argues that in a recent Swedish vaccine trial, there was no benefit of the acellular vaccine over the whole-cell vaccine as to efficacy nor as to "the frequency of serious adverse events, including hypotonic hyporesponsive episodes".*
> *Local side-effects are generally admitted. They consist of redness and swelling.*

Systemic reactions, however, also occur. Examples are fever, drowsiness, irritability, prolonged, high-pitched crying and seizures.

In one study there was no difference with the old vaccine with respect to fussiness, antipyretic use, drowsiness, or anorexia. Uberall noticed convulsions within three days of vaccination occurred in 1/15,912 doses in DTaP recipients.

Persistent inconsolable crying, a sure sign of brain inflammation, was present in 1/497 doses.

High fever (<40.5°C) was observed in 1/16,239 doses. One hypotonic-hyporesponsive episode was observed in 4,273 DTaP recipients.

Fever, injection site redness, swelling, and pain increased in prevalence with increasing numbers of injections. "For children receiving DTaP as a fourth dose, injection site redness and swelling occurred more frequently in DtaP primed than in DTwP-primed children".

By this time, professionals began to be concerned that parents were being falsely accused of SBS after a possible vaccine injury. Their main concern was that the DTP and some brands of the DTaP, alongside other vaccines in use, included the preservative thimerosal. Thimerosal is a mercury-containing organic compound used as a preservative in many vaccines and is said to help prevent potentially life-threatening contamination with harmful microbes. This preservative is 49.6 percent *ethyl mercury, a highly toxic poison that is geno-toxic and neurotoxic.* Some professionals say it collects in the brain and organs like the kidneys. It is also said to interfere with our DNA and can affect our brain and immune system. It also is believed to affect the retina. Although not used in all vaccines (for example, it is not used in measles-mumps-rubella or chickenpox vaccines), it was originally used in the manufacture of many early vaccines and has been since the early 1930s. It has been frequently linked to neurological problems in children. In 1999, thimerosal was removed from many childhood vaccines because the Public Health Service agencies and the AAP (American Academy of Pediatrics) recommended that *thimerosal* be *taken out of vaccines* as a precautionary measure. However, it still remains in a few today.

One professional who grew increasingly concerned about the use of thimerosal in vaccines was Lisa Blakemore-Brown, a psychologist, author, and expert in autism. Blakemore-Brown has been particularly worried about the issues surrounding false accusations of child abuse, including accusations of MSBP/FII/SBS/SIDS, especially in cases where a child has had an adverse reaction to a vaccine. She has voiced her concerns on many occasions, both to the government and through the media, stating on her blog 'Thimerosal Thoughts' in 2007[129]:

> *Recently a new paper was published by Hey and Bacon on the sensitive subject of how many mothers might have murdered their babies who died of 'cot death'. Yet a known and well researched link (under a heavy cloak of commercial secrecy) is that of an adverse reaction to some vaccinations but this is never mentioned.*
>
> *Over the years there have been many forms of spin and shifting sands of blame and counter blame but none so deeply distressing as the accusation that a mother has killed her child. What stands out when mothers are accused is that adverse reactions to vaccine are routinely NEVER included in the differential diagnosis. This is deeply worrying, as it is a well known form of iatrogenic abuse. However rare, it happens, but if we do not acknowledge that it happens, and could have happened to the child in question, then as all other possibilities fall away, the mother stands accused.*

She is totally correct in my opinion, and this is a question I have asked myself on many occasions: Why are vaccines never considered as a possibility for the death of the many children who die within hours or days of multiple vaccines?

From the evidence found, whether the DTP or the DTaP is given to infants, a picture has emerged showing similar adverse reactions have been reported throughout history, in particular, persistent high-pitched crying and convulsions, leading in some cases to severe disability or death.

DTP/DTaP Ingredients - Dawn Winkler -Vaccine Ingredients [130]

DTP
Diphtheria and Tetanus Toxoids and Pertussis Vaccine Adsorbed
SmithKline Beecham Pharmaceuticals
1-800-366-8900 ext. 5231
produced using aluminum phosphate, formaldehyde, ammonium sulfate, washed sheep red blood cells, glycerol, sodium chloride, thimerosal
medium: porcine (pig) pancreatic hydrolysate of casein

Acel-Immune
DTaP
Diphtheria and Tetanus Toxoids and Acellular Pertussis Vaccine Adsorbed
Lederle Laboratories
1-800-934-5556
produced using formaldehyde, thimerosal, aluminum hydroxide, aluminum phosphate, polysorbate 80, gelatin

Some manufacturers have now removed thimerosal.
Source: 1997 Physicians' Desk Reference
Toll-free numbers can be called to obtain product inserts.
This is a representative, not a comprehensive, list of the various types of vaccines.[131]

Haemophilus Influenzae Type B Vaccine

Moving swiftly on, we look at the Hib or Haemophilus influenzae type b vaccination, which was first introduced to the vaccine schedule in the early 1990s. This vaccine is given to babies to prevent them from contracting Haemophilus influenzae type b. Hib is not believed to have any relationship to the flu and instead is a serious bacterial infection that can cause meningitis, pneumonia, swelling of the throat, and other disease complications.

Although serious adverse reactions have been reported after the Hib vaccine, it has been difficult to establish which vaccine is responsible for the reactions being reported, as Hib is often given alongside other vaccines. The National Vaccine Information Centre (NVIC)[132] reports the following:

> *Haemophilus Influenza Type B Vaccine (HIB)*
>
> *Reported common reactions to Hib vaccine include fever and pain and swelling at injection site. Rash, hives, irritability, restless sleep, prolonged crying; diarrhea, vomiting, loss of appetite, convulsions, collapse/shock, and Guillain-Barre syndrome have also been reported. Some of the studies used to evaluate the reactivity of Hib vaccine were complicated by the fact that Hib vaccine was given simultaneously with DPT an OPV vaccine. When a reaction occurred, it was difficult to determine which vaccines were responsible for the reaction.*
>
> *In 1994, the Institute of Medicine concluded that there is compelling scientific evidence that vaccination with earlier versions of the Hib vaccine resulted in early onset of Hib disease in children over 18 months of age. Apparently, the early Hib vaccines caused children, who had been recently vaccinated, to be immune suppressed for at least 7 days after vaccination.*

If children become immune suppressed, it leaves them open to catch other illnesses. If they are being vaccinated with a vaccine that suppresses their immune system, then surely they are more susceptible to illnesses like meningitis, one of the illnesses that the Hib vaccine is given to protect them against. This, of course, is also true for encephalitis, which is an inflammation of the brain caused by infection.

In the list of facts on encephalitis that is on the Encephalitis Society website[133] it says that inflammation is usually caused by an inappropriate autoimmune response to infection.

- Encephalitis is inflammation of the brain.
- **Inflammation is usually caused by infection or an inappropriate auto-immune response to infection.**

- The incidence is reported as 7.4/100,000 (based on U.S. statistics).
- Anyone can become ill with encephalitis, at any age.
- The inflammation can damage nerve cells resulting in "acquired brain injury."
- Compared to other infectious diseases, encephalitis has a high mortality rate.

If a child's immune system is suppressed by the Hib vaccine, as suggested by the NVIC when they say, *"the early Hib vaccines caused children, who had been recently vaccinated, to be immune suppressed for at least 7 days after vaccination,"* then it could cause the child to contract an infection that leads the brain to become inflamed, causing him or her to die without warning, suffering SIDS as an end result. SIDS is a possible reaction, stated by NVIC[132] further on in their information :

> *The conjugate Hib vaccines now being used are thought to be more quickly effective, leaving children less vulnerable to Hib disease shortly after vaccination. However, the IOM report stated that "Because immunization with Hib vaccines may lead to a transient decrease in protective antibody levels, unimmunized children at increased risk of colonization (household or day-care contact with individuals with recent cases of Hib infection) may require special [protective] measures." One Hib vaccine manufacturer states, "There have been rare reports to the Vaccine Adverse Events Reporting System (VAERS) of Hib disease following full primary immunization."*
>
> *Because either no studies or too few studies have ever been conducted to investigate Hib vaccine reactions, the IOM could not make a determination about whether Hib vaccine causes transverse myelitis, Guillain-Barre syndrome, thrombocytopenia, anaphylaxis and **sudden infant death syndrome.***

Pharmacist Heidi White wrote a paper in 1999[134] linking the Hib vaccination to asthma. She explained how different studies in rats, mice, and guinea pigs supported this:

a) A nasal Hib vaccine has been shown to stimulate Th1 and Th2 cells in mice.[3] If the Th2 side of the immune system is over stimulated, then this can increase the risk of asthma and allergy.

b) Hib vaccination in rats has been shown to enhance histamine levels with a corresponding increase in the number of eosinophils.[4-7] Eosinophils (white blood cells, used to fight infection) will proliferate and accumulate in the airways under stimulation by interleukin-5 (IL-5), a cytokine produced by Th2 cells. Eosinophil accumulation is also evident in the dermis of the skin seen in people with atopic dermatitis (eczema).

c) Hib vaccination in rats has been shown to cause increased bronchoconstriction in response to histamine, possibly due to an increased reactivity of the para-sympathetic/cholinergic pathways.[7,8]

*d) Studies in guinea-pigs have shown that Hib vaccination may impair the beta (b) 2-adrenergic system by causing a blocking or desensitization of b 2 receptors, or by reducing the number of b 2 receptors in the lung.[9-13] Inhibition of b receptors can lead to increased bronchoconstriction. It is thought that the polysaccharide component of the bacterial cell wall may be responsible for this effect.[14] **HibTitre** vaccine contains purified polysaccharide (PRP), from the capsule of the Hib bacteria, which is linked to a diphtheria carrier protein. **PedvaxHIB** vaccine contains PRP linked to a meningococcal protein.*

However, she finishes her article by adding that at that time no human studies had been carried out to support her theory.

It is highly probable that her studies are correct, as some manufacturers use yeast as an ingredient of the Hib vaccine and an allergy to yeast is known to cause asthma and breathing difficulties in some children. Severe asthma attacks can and do lead to death, so therefore it is possible that babies have died after a combination of vaccines including the Hib vaccine because they have reacted to the yeast component of the vaccine.

Lauren DiMiceli and associates[135] carried out a study using the Vaccine Adverse Events Reporting System database as a tool. They reported that they found that some children have reacted adversely to the yeast used in vaccinations. The problems they found were mostly linked to the Hep B vaccine, which has been known to be given to babies alongside the Hib vaccine. If two vaccines containing yeast were used simultaneously, one could assume that any problem an infant with a yeast allergy may face would be twofold in magnitude. The abstract to their study reads:

> *The preparation of recombinant hepatitis B vaccines involves using cellular cultures of Saccharomyces cerevisiae, otherwise known as baker's yeast. Prior to vaccine licensure, clinical trials were performed to address whether residual yeast proteins in the vaccines could induce anaphylaxis, including testing for IgE anti-yeast antibody levels. 1–2% of subjects had anti-yeast IgE antibodies before immunization, but demonstrated no significant rise in IgE after HBV. We searched reports in the Vaccine Adverse Event Reporting System (VAERS) for those that mentioned a history of allergy to yeast and then reviewed the adverse events described in these reports for potential anaphylactic reactions. Probable anaphylaxis was defined as the presence of one or more dermatologic symptoms and one or more respiratory, gastrointestinal, or cardiovascular symptoms with onset within 4 h of Hepatitis B vaccination. Possible anaphylaxis was defined in one of two ways: (1) cases that described dermatologic or respiratory symptoms (but not both) occurring within 4 h of vaccination; or (2) cases that described one or more dermatologic and/or respiratory symptoms occurring 4–12 h post vaccination. Among the 107 reports of pre-existing "yeast allergies," 11 reports described probable or possible anaphylaxis after HBV. Four additional cases were described after other vaccines. The majority of vaccines who met the case definitions and had a history of yeast allergies were female, ages ranged from 10 to 64, and symptom onset ranged from 15 min to 5 h after vaccination. No deaths were reported. The small number of reports to VAERS may be partly due to health care professionals observing current contraindications by not vaccinating yeast sensitive individuals. Nevertheless, yeast associated anaphylaxis after HBV in sensitized patients appears to be a rare event.*

The National Vaccine Information Centre also stated that it is difficult to identify what adverse reactions can be attributed to the Hib vaccine, if any, as it is usual for Hib to be given with other vaccines. These are the reactions so far reported:

Haemophilus Influenza Type B Vaccine (HIB)

Reported common reactions to Hib vaccine include fever and pain and swelling at injection site. Rash, hives, irritability, restless sleep, prolonged crying; diarrhea, vomiting, loss of appetite, convulsions, collapse/shock, and Guillain-Barre syndrome have also been reported.

As I have shown, sudden infant death has been reported after a Hib vaccine; however, again, this is usually when it is given as part of a combination of vaccines.

The National Vaccine Information Centre stated:

In 1994, the Institute of Medicine concluded that there is compelling scientific evidence that vaccination with earlier versions of the Hib vaccine resulted in early onset of Hib disease in children over 18 months of age. Apparently, the early Hib vaccines caused children, who had been recently vaccinated, to be immune suppressed for at least 7 days after vaccination.

The conjugate Hib vaccines now being used are thought to be more quickly effective, leaving children less vulnerable to Hib disease shortly after vaccination. However, the IOM report stated that "Because immunization with Hib vaccines may lead to a transient decrease in protective antibody levels, unimmunized children at increased risk of colonization (household or day-care contact with individuals with recent cases of Hib infection) may require special [protective] measures." One Hib vaccine manufacturer states, "There have been rare reports to the Vaccine Adverse Events Reporting System (VAERS) of Hib disease following full primary immunization."

Because either no studies or too few studies have ever been conducted to investigate Hib vaccine reactions, the IOM could *not make a determination about whether Hib vaccine causes transverse myelitis, Guillain-Barre syndrome, thrombocytopenia, anaphylaxis and **sudden infant death syndrome.***

There have been quite a few reports of parents accused of having shaken their babies, SBS, after the Hib vaccination has been administered, but these have been where the baby has had a number of vaccines at the same time. Viera Scheibner Phd[136] has been convinced for many years that there is a definite link between vaccination and the sudden deterioration of a baby (very often premature babies) resulting in brain injury, even death, after multiple vaccines. We can see from her paper the SBS cases that have been reported are after all the vaccines used in the five-in-one vaccines have been administered. She says:

> *Some time ago I started getting requests from lawyers or the accused parents themselves for expert reports. A close study of the history of these cases revealed something distinctly sinister: in every single case, the symptoms appeared shortly after the baby's vaccinations.*
>
> *While investigating the personal medical history of these babies based on the care-giver's diaries and medical records, I quickly established that these babies were given one or more of the series of so-called routine shots—hepatitis B, DPT (diphtheria, pertussis, tetanus), polio and HIB (Haemophilus influenzae type B—shortly before they developed symptoms of illness resulting in serious brain damage or death.*
>
> *The usual scenario is that a baby is born and does well initially. At the usual age of about two months it is administered the first series of vaccines as above. (Sometimes a hepatitis B injection is given shortly after birth while the mother and child are still in hospital. However, a great number of babies now die within days or within two to four weeks of birth after hepatitis B vaccination, as documented by the records of the VAERS [Vaccine Adverse Event Reporting System] in the USA.) So, the baby stops progressing, starts deteriorating, and usually develops signs of respiratory tract infection. Then comes the second and third injections, and tragedy strikes: the child may cry intensely and inconsolably, may stop feeding*

properly, vomit, have difficulty swallowing, become irritable, stop sleeping, and may develop convulsions with accelerating progressive deterioration of its condition and mainly its brain function.

This deterioration may be fast, or may slowly inch in until the parents notice that some-thing is very wrong with their child and then rush it to the doctor or hospital. Interestingly, they are invariably asked when the baby was immunised. On learning that the baby was indeed "immunised", the parents may be reassured that its symptoms will all clear up. They are sent home with the advice, "Give your baby Panadol". If they persist in considering the baby's reaction serious, they may be labelled as anxious parents or trouble-makers. So the parents go home, and the child remains in a serious condition or dies.

Until recently, the vaccine death would have just been la-belled "sudden infant death", particularly if the symptoms and pathological findings were minimal. However, nowadays, with an alarmingly increasing frequency, the parents (or at least one of them, usually the father) may be accused of shaking the baby to death. The accused may even "confess" to shaking the baby, giving the reason, for example, that having found the baby lying still and not breathing and/or with a glazed look in its eyes, they shook it gently—as is only natural—in their attempt to revive it. Sometimes, ironically, they save the baby's life, only to be accused of causing the internal injuries that made the baby stop breathing in the first place, and which in fact were already present when they shook the baby to revive it.

No matter what the parents say or do, everything is con-strued against them. If they are crying and emotional, they will be accused of showing signs of guilt. If they manage to remain composed and unemotional, they will be called calculating and controlling—and guilty because of that.

Sadly the above is becoming more common and may be a result of the vast quantity of vaccinations given at the same time, or due to babies being allergic to one or more of a vaccine's contents.

Hib Haemophilus Influenza Type B Ingredients

Haemophilus—Influenza B Connaught Laboratories, 800-822-2463
* Haemophilus influenza Type B, polyribosylribitol phosphate ammonium sulfate, formalin, and sucrose

HiB Titer—Haemophilus Influenza B Wyeth-Ayerst, 800-934-5556
* haemophilus influenza B, polyribosylribitol phosphate, yeast, ammonium sulfate, thimerosal, and chemically defined yeast-based medium

Hib Hib saccharides cultured on cows' brains; CRM protein; neomycin; streptomycin; polymyxin B.

Ingredients listed on Rense.com[137]

Polio Vaccine

The polio vaccine is given to protect children against the polio virus. Polio, or poliomyelitis, is an acute viral infection that involves the gastrointestinal tract and occasionally the central nervous system. Years ago it was this virus that caused many thousands of cases of paralysis worldwide. The polio vaccine comes in two forms, the IPV or OPV. The IPV is the inactivated poliovirus vaccine, and the OPV is the live, oral poliovirus vaccine; however, the OPV is no longer recommended.

The first ever polio vaccines were given during the 1950s. The vaccine was developed at the University of Pittsburgh by Dr. Jonas Salk, who had begun his medical research career studying immunology. There were problems reported from the beginning. Bonnie A. Maybury Okonek and associates write[138]:

> *In 1947, while at the University of Pittsburgh, he began his research on poliovirus. His research was greatly helped in 1949, when a method of growing poliovirus in cell culture, instead of having to use primarily monkeys for research, was*

discovered. Salk needed to find a way to process the viruses so that they were less infectious, before using them in a vaccine. In 1952, Salk was the first to develop a successful vaccine using a mixture of the three types of virus, grown in monkey kidney cultures. He developed a process using formalin, a chemical that inactivated the whole virus.

What followed was massive testing of the vaccine in clinical trials in the United States and parts of Canada, begun in 1954. The scope of the trials was unprecedented in medical history. The results were dramatic. Cases of polio fell spectacularly in the vaccinated test groups. In 1955, the government quickly granted permission for the vaccine to be distributed to the children of our country.

But, there was a problem with the original Salk vaccine. The vaccine actually induced 260 cases of poliomyelitis, including 10 deaths.

The problem was, even though other versions of the vaccine were manufactured, the safety issues surrounding adverse reactions and efficiency persisted. Governments around the world continued to hype up the vaccine's benefits, encouraging more people to be vaccinated, stating that the vaccine was a safe vaccine; however, the medical world was saying quite the opposite. Below are a few examples.

These two examples have been taken from a book written by Eleanor Mc|Bean , The Poisoned Needle – Suppressed Facts About Vaccination

The Hidden Dangers in Polio Vaccine [139]

Dr. Ritchie Russell of the Department of Neurology, Radcliffe Infirmary Oxford, said, "When poliomyelitis is precipitated by inoculation the natural defences of the nervous system seem to be ineffective, and nearly all such illnesses develop into a paralytic form of the disease affecting especially the limb used for the injection." (Lancet, May 21, 1955, p. 1071)

An editorial in the Lancet (weekly Medical Journal, April 23, 1955) comments: "If it is found that, contrary to Salk's

*hopes antibody levels cannot be maintained without a suc-cession of booster doses, then a serious problem will arise. Will it be necessary to give injections every year; and, if so, for how long would they be given? ... **If injections are given regularly for several years to millions of children the risk of allergic reactions to monkey kidney tissue will become increasingly grave.***"

The Manchester Guardian *(April 15, 1955) stated, "One of Britain's greatest physiologists said to-day that if it means that a child should be re-inoculated at frequent intervals with a preparation derived from monkey kidneys it is terrifying in its possibilities. Among them is the risk of the child's develop-ing sensitivity to some of the ingredients of the vaccine." The editor of the Lancet (June 11, 1955, p. 1207) emphasized this further when he wrote: "**In addition to the possibility of producing the very disease the vaccine is used to prevent, there is a risk, of unknown dimensions, that repeated injection of a vaccine prepared from monkey kidney may eventually sensitize the child in some harmful way.**"*

Sadly the deaths after the vaccine continued as well.

A PARTIAL LIST OF DEATHS FROM SALK VACCINE
Susan Pierce (age 7), Pocatello, Idaho, died April 27, 1955
Ronald Fitzgerald (age 4), Oakland, Calif., died April 27, 1955
Allen Davis Jr. (age 2), New Orleans, La., died May 4, 1955
Janet Kincaid (age 7), Moscow, Idaho, died May 1, 1955
Danny Eggers (age 6), Idaho Falls, Idaho, died May 10, 1955
Reference as above [139]

Another fact that slowly emerged was that the polio vaccine was proving to be inefficient. Studies showed that the duration of the vaccine's protection, if any, was short lived. This was pointed out in the editorial in the *Lancet* (weekly Medical Journal, April 23, 1955).

As with each of the other vaccines that I have identified, the polio vaccine has also been associated with cases involving SBS accusations, including Alan Raymond Yurko, who was found guilty of aggravated child abuse and first-degree murder after the death of his infant son, Alan Joseph. Louise Mclean[140] reports:

> *Baby Alan was born prematurely at 35 weeks on 16th September, 1997. His mother Francine had suffered health problems during the pregnancy including gestational diabetes, urinary and vaginal infections, E coli infection, had been treated with antibiotics and had also lost significant weight during her pregnancy.*
>
> *The infant weighing 5 lb. 8 oz at birth was suffering respiratory distress, placed in intensive care and given antibiotics. As well as showing decreased muscle tone and activity, the baby developed jaundice, severe hypoxia (deficiency of oxygen in the tissues), acidosis, dehydration, hypoglycemia and reduced renal function. Despite continuing to experience respiratory problems with grunting and breathlessness, continuing jaundice, wind, painful bowel movements and bloated stomach, on 11th November 1997 Baby Alan received a cocktail of six vaccines. These were diptheria, tetanus, pertussis, haemaphilus influenza B, oral polio and hepatitis B.*
>
> *Approximately 10 days later, Baby Alan exhibited lethargy, irritability, no appetite, fever and developed a high pitched cry. By 24th November, 1997, Baby Alan began wheezing, vomiting and stopped breathing. Alan rushed him to Florida's Orlando hospital, giving mouth to mouth resuscitation all the way. On arrival at the hospital the baby had turned blue. Somehow Alan pushed his way in and watched doctors insert a large tube down the baby's throat pumping air into his stomach, which blew up like a beach ball. A doctor shouted 'wrong tube, wrong tube!' This procedure was repeated, again with Baby Alan's stomach ballooning up. They then put a huge needle in his chest and got the shock pads.*
>
> *Finally he started to breathe again. Alan and Francine were ecstatic. The doctors decided the baby must be moved to a larger hospital with a special breathing machine because they thought he was septic.*
>
> *It was at this second hospital that baby Alan eventually died. Alan and Francine were not allowed in to see what was*

happening to him but waited and waited outside. A doctor came out and told them quite simply that Alan was going to die, that he had broken ribs and his brain was bleeding.

Viera Scheibner, PhD, in an article I mentioned previously,[136] said:

While investigating the personal medical history of these babies based on the care-giver's diaries and medical records, I quickly established that these babies were given one or more of the series of so-called routine shots—hepatitis B, DPT (diphtheria, pertussis, tetanus), polio and HIB (Haemophilus influenzae type B—shortly before they developed symptoms of illness resulting in serious brain damage or death.

There is very little evidence on accusations of SBS surrounding any one of these vaccinations individually; however, when these vaccines are given as a combination of separate vaccines simultaneously, problems begin to emerge.

Polio Vaccine Ingredients

IPOL Connaught Laboratories, 800-822-2463
* 3 types of polio viruses neomycin, streptomycin, and polymyxin B formaldehyde, and 2-phenoxyethenol continuous line of monkey kidney cells

Orimune—Oral Polio Wyeth-Ayerst, 800-934-5556
* 3 types of polio viruses, attenuated neomycin, streptomycin sorbitol monkey kidney cells and calf serum

Three strains of polio virus; formaldehyde; aluminum phosphate or aluminum hydroxide; neomycin, streptomycin and polymyxin B (antibiotics); 2-phenoxyethanol (a preservative); medium 199, which contains polysorbate 80 (an emulsifier); cultured on monkey kidney cells or calf fetus tissue. The inactivated (injectable) polio vaccine is cultivated on vero cells (African green monkey kidney cells).

Vaccine ingredients listed on Rense.com[137]

Hep B Vaccine

The hepatitis B vaccine is a vaccine that has been developed for the prevention of hepatitis B infection. The vaccine contains one of the what is called *'viral envelope proteins'*, hepatitis B surface antigen or (HBsAg). It is produced by using yeast cells, into which the genetic code for HBsAg has been inserted. A course of three of the doses of the vaccine are usually given, with the second dose given approximately one month after the first dose and the third dose given approximately six months after the first dose. Afterward, an immune system antibody to HBsAg is established in the bloodstream. This antibody is known as *anti-HBsAg*. This antibody and immune system memory then provides us with an immunity to hepatitis B infection. The first Hep B vaccine became available in 1981.

The hepatitis B vaccine has been a troubled vaccine from the onset. In 1981, the first Hep B vaccine came into use, but the original vaccine was discontinued in 1990 because it was an "inactivated" type of vaccine that involved the collection of blood from hepatitis B virus-infected (HBsAg-positive) donors. The pooled blood was said to be subjected to multiple steps to inactive the viral particles, including formaldehyde and heat treatment (or "pasteurization"). The vaccine was by Merck Pharmaceuticals and manufactured as "Heptavax," and was the first commercial hepatitis B virus vaccine.

In the United States in 1996, it was reported that there were 872 serious adverse events in children under the age of fourteen years who had been vaccinated with hepatitis B vaccine. Out of these, forty-eight children were said to have died as a result of having the Hep B vaccine. When these figures are compared to the lower figure of 279 children under the age of fourteen years who contracted Hepatitis B infection in the same year, you have to wonder whether the vaccine was proving more dangerous than the threat of contracting the actual disease.

In fact, according to Dr. Gregory Damato,[141] there were 24,775 adverse reactions reported to the Vaccine Adverse Events Reporting System (VAERS) from 1990 through 1999. These include 439 deaths and 9,673 emergency room visits. There were also reports of arthritis, skin disorders, compromised immunity and autoimmune disease, neurological damage; vision loss and rare eye disorders, such as optic neuritis and epitheliopathy; blood disorders, diabetes, damage to liver and kidneys, severe vomiting, and diarrhea. We must at this stage remind ourselves that VAERS is a US-based system only. If these were the figures for just the United States, one must think of the wider picture.

The vaccine is currently given to a baby at birth, although many see this as unwise; unless a baby is known to be at risk from hepatitis B, this could put the baby at immediate risk from adverse vaccine reactions. As hepatitis B can only be transmitted through direct contact with infectious blood, semen, and/or body fluids through sex, sharing needles, or infected mother to newborn, it is highly unlikely that the majority of babies born will be infected. Many experts see the vaccination of all children at birth as a step too far.

The vaccine is cultivated in yeast. BioPharm International[142] says this is because:

> *Yeasts are distinguished by a growing track record as expression platforms for the production of pharmaceuticals. Commercially available, yeast-derived, recombinant pharmaceuticals include, among others, insulin, the anti-coagulant hirudin, interferon-alpha-2a, and various vaccines against the hepatitis B virus and papillomavirus infections. The vaccines are produced in either baker's yeast (Saccharomyces cerevisiae), or the methylotrophic species Hansenula polymorpha and Pichia pastoris. In this article, we focus on a production process for hepatitis B vaccines in methylotrophs. Methylotrophs provide highly balanced production of both the membrane and the protein component of a recombinant viral particle. A brief outlook is given for the development of yeast strains designed for the production of other vaccine candidates.*

However, this can cause some children to react very severely to the vaccine, especially if they have an allergy to yeast. The Hepatitis B Foundation[143] states, *"The vaccine may not be recommended for those with documented yeast allergies or a history of an adverse reaction to the vaccine."* The main problem with this statement is that if these vaccines are given to a baby on the day they are born, no one knows if: (a) the baby has an allergy to yeast, or b) whether the child has an allergy to any of the other of the vaccine ingredients.

One doctor, who is pro vaccine, Dr. Bernadine Healy, has also expressed concern about infants receiving hep B shots. She, alongside other medical experts, worries about the necessity of exposing infants to this vaccine and it's potential side effects at such an early age unless they are at risk from contracting the disease. She told the CBS News that[144] *"most infants have no direct contact with body fluids of someone infected with hepatitis B, so what's the rush in exposing them to the series of vaccinations?"*

According to the CBS News report,[144] a special Vaccine Court ruled in 2009 that the hep B vaccine was responsible for one woman becoming ill with an MS-type illness after she was vaccinated. The woman later died. According to the Vaccine Court:

> *"There is a logical sequence of cause and effect in petitioner's having received the vaccination and then experiencing optic neuritis, the first symptom of her Devic's Disease, a variant of MS. As discussed, the onset after vaccination is appropriate to prove causation, whether the onset is 18 days or two months after vaccination ... Not only did decedent have a vaccine injury, but also her death was vaccine-related."*
>
> *This decision, like others in Vaccine Court, appears to contradict the government's official position. In 2002, the Institute of Medicine (Dr. Healy is a member, but does not agree with all of the group's views) stated: "The epidemiological evidence favors rejection of a causal relationship between the hepatitis B vaccine in adults and multiple sclerosis. Because of the lack of epidemiological data on conditions other than MS in adults, the committee recommends further attention in the form of research and communication. However, the committee does not recommend that national and federal vaccine advisory*

bodies review the hepatitis B vaccine on the basis of concerns about demyelinating disorders."

The news report says that according to the government's statistics, at least 123 people who have filed cases in Vaccine Court have been paid compensation by the government for injuries or death relating to their hep B vaccine.

An article in the *American Chronicle*[145] explains that in one paper available online, Dr. Marc Girard, a specialist in the side effects of drugs and commissioned as a medical expert by French courts in the criminal investigation into the introduction of universal hepatitis B vaccination in France, suggests that even in high-endemic countries, the risk/benefit ratio of what he describes as "this unusually toxic vaccine" must be carefully reassessed. Regarding the health situation in the UK, Dr. Girard says the conclusion not to vaccinate is obvious. France was the first country to implement universal hepatitis B vaccination in 1994.

It has been reported that while much evidence is embargoed by the French courts, Dr. Marc Girard has also been able to publish a scientific review of the unembargoed evidence of the vaccine's hazards Autoimmun Rev 2005; 4: 96–100[146]. Dr. Girard shows in his paper that the French health authorities suppressed studies demonstrating serious risks. His new paper reviews the various mechanisms likely to account for the biological plausibility of autoimmune disorders, such as demyelinating diseases, and other hazards of this vaccine.

Legal and ethical concerns also arise over the British Medical Association's (BMA) recommendation because those at high risk from the hepatitis B virus are not usually infants, but instead are adults engaging in unsafe sex and intravenous drug abusers. There is no clear individual clinical benefit of universal hepatitis B vaccination. The duration of any protective effect is also uncertain, and this is worrying. What does seem apparent however, is that the vaccination carries with it possible risks of numerous chronic autoimmune disorder. These include Guillain-Barre syndrome, lupus, rheumatism, blood disorders, and chronic fatigue.

The British Medical Association is suggesting that a child can get infected with hep B by biting and shared toys, shared toothbrushes and razors, and mother-to-child transmission during birth. Dr Girard said:

> *The BMA's recommendation is a surprising and unexpected change of heart given the scathing public scepticism in the British Medical Journal in 1996 to a pharmaceutical company promotion advocating universal infant hepatitis B vaccination (BMJ 1996; 313: 825). It is all the more surprising because whilst the risk factors for babies have changed little, there is now impressive evidence that for a preventive measure, hepatitis B vaccine is remarkable for the frequency, variety and severity of complications from its use. The toxicity of this vaccine is so unusual that, even if crucial data are regrettably concealed or covered by Court order, scientific evidence is already far higher than normally needed to justify severe restrictive measures.*

Clearly much controversy surrounds the safety of hep B vaccination.

Hepatitis B Vaccine Ingredients

Energix-B
Recombinant Hepatitis B, GlaxoSmithKline, 800-366-8900 x5231
* genetic sequence of the hepatitis B virus that codes for the surface antigen (HbSAg), cloned into GMO yeast, aluminum hydroxide, and thimerosal

Chapter 8

The Five In One Vaccines - The Pharmaceutical Industries Cauldron

DTaP/HIB/IPV or DtaP/HIB/HepB or Five-in-One Combination Vaccines

There are two different types of five-in-one combination vaccines in use today. These are DTaP/HIB/IPV or DtaP/HIB/HepB. One of the five-in-one combination vaccines to go onto the market is Pentacel; it was introduced to the vaccination schedule for children in 1997. Pentacel is a five-in-one combination vaccine combining DTaP, HiB, and polio. It is the first DTaP-based combination vaccine that also included polio and HiB vaccine components. Similar five-in-one vaccines, such as Pediarix and Pediacel, were also introduced. However, controversy has arisen over the use of the Pentacel vaccine because the polio portion of this vaccine is grown on the MRC-5 cell line derived from human fetuses. This is said to have particularly raised concerns of the Catholic community, as they are said to feel that it is unethical to use vaccines from cell lines. In an article entitled "Alternatives to Vaccines Made from Aborted Babies," Catherine Williams[147] gives these reasons:

- *If abortion is immoral then profiting from it must also be immoral.*
- *The unborn child was unable to give consent for its body parts to be used, so it is therefore disrespectful to the dead. This is different from an adult donating a body part*

> *such as a kidney (as one vaccine manufacturer claimed)*
> *because the adult must always have given consent.*

- *Some would argue that the fetal tissues would just go to waste if they were not used but this excuse was not accepted at the Nuremberg trials of scientists who used body parts from concentration camp victims. This abuse of the child's body only compounds the injustice of the original abortion, even if the vaccine producers were in no way connected to the abortion.*

- *Use of this vaccine implies acceptance of the legality of abortion, and does nothing to discourage the use of fetal parts or cell lines in vaccine manufacture or other branches of medicine, or to encourage research into other materials.*

- *We believe it would be wrong to give our children a vaccine which we would not use on ourselves when they are too young to decide for themselves. We have taught them that abortion is wrong it would therefore be inconsistent to give them the vaccine.*

- *Some people do not consider the manufacture of vaccines from animals to be ethical. Such people will not be able to accept any viral vaccine, since a virus has to be grown on living cells. However we do not take this view.*

Straightaway a large number of adverse reactions began to be reported from around the world. The Deccan Herald[148] reported that an article in the *British Medical Journal* (BMJ) reported that the five-in-one vaccine that had been recommended in India by the National Technical Advisory Group on Immunization actually killed children in Sri Lanka and Bhutan. This five-in-one vaccine was the vaccine that included the hep B component as opposed to the polio.

A report in LankaNewspapers.com[149] stated the following:

> *The report by a group, including paediatricians, professors, health activists and a former Indian health secretary, cautions against the introduction of the five-in-one vaccine that combines antigens against five diseases—diphtheria, pertussis,*

tetanus (DPT), hepatitis B and Haemophilus Influenzae type B (HIB)—in a single shot.

> *Our article describes how the World Health Organisation (WHO), in an elaborate cover-up, changed its own criteria for classifying adverse effects to say the vaccine was not responsible for the deaths in Sri Lanka, Jacob Puliyel, head of paediatrics at St Stephen s Hospital in Delhi and key author, told IANS."*

> *Former union health secretary K.B. Saxena, professors of community health in Jawaharlal Nehru University in Delhi Debabar Banerji, Imrana Qadeer and Ritu Priya, co-conveners of All India Drug Action Network Mira Shiva and Gopal Dabade and former adviser in finance ministry N.J. Kurian are the other authors of the report.*

> *The authors point out that the pentavalent vaccine was withdrawn in Sri Lanka in April 2008 after 25 serious adverse reactions that included five deaths and Bhutan stopped its use within two months of introduction in July 2009 after eight deaths.*

> *Bhutan has so far resisted pressure from WHO to restart immunisation but Sri Lanka reintroduced the vaccine this year after a WHO expert panel, which investigated the events, declared that the vaccine was unlikely to have caused the deaths.*

> *The panel, however, could not conclusively attribute the deaths to any other cause.*

The Vaccine Risk Awareness Network (VRAN), an organization based in Canada that is a public information and resource group that supplies information about risks and potential side effects of vaccines, also reported problems. In an e-mail, Edda West from VRAN[150] said:

> *Here in Canada, we didn't hear a peep in the media when Aventis Pasteur's 5 in 1 vaccine (Pentacel) was introduced across the board and injected into most Canadian babies starting in 1997.*

> *Although we can be grateful that thimerosal is no longer in the vaccine (except perhaps for trace amounts used in the*

manufacturing process which apparently they don't have to disclose), it has been replaced with <u>2-phenoxyethanol</u>, a main ingredient in anti-freeze. You'd need to check the ingredients list to determine whether this is also being used in the U.K. version of the 5 in 1 vaccine. We've not been able to find any data showing that it is safe to inject infants with 2-phenoxyethanol or anti-freeze for that matter. Our understanding is that they were unable to continue using thimerosal, not because of safety concerns to babies, but because the inactivated polio viruses in Pentacel vaccine are altered by thimerosal, hence the need to switch to another preservative. Some sources state that 2-phenoxyethanol is a 'protoplasmic poison'. No matter how many vaccines your David Salisbury and Paul Offit in the U.S. think babies can handle, the bottom line is they are still being injected with toxic substances.

Canadian infants have been the main test market for this vaccine these past 7 years, and based on this large experiment, Aventis is aiming to have it licensed for use in the U.S. either in 2004 or 05. Undoubtedly licensing in other countries is pending as well.

There has been a HUGE increase in anaphylaxis disorders following the widespread use of the 5 in 1 vaccine and its precursor Penta (4 in one plus Hib). Attached is a letter from a parent whose child developed anaphylaxis following injection with Penta, the precursor to Pentacel—it took her over a year to get a list of reactions to the lot numbers of vaccine her boy was injected with. Of course we have no idea how many lot numbers were issued in all, or how many children overall were vaccinated during the course of this experiment before they created its progeny, the 5 in 1 vaccine trademarked Pentacel in Canada.

Best wishes,

Edda West,

VRAN—Vaccination Risk Awareness Network Inc.

VRAN has certainly raised some interesting questions. It is of particular interest that there has been a huge rise in anaphylaxic disorders, especially if looked at in relation to parents being falsely accused of SBS. In the paper "Shaken Baby/Impact Syndrome:

Flawed Concepts and Misdiagnoses" by Dr. Harold E. Buttram,[151] this is referenced in studies involving mice and the pertussis vaccine, which is a vaccine used in the five-in-one combination.

> *It is noteworthy that vaccines such as pertussis have been used to induce allergic encephalomyelitis in laboratory animals since 1973, (44) characterized by brain swelling and hemorrhages similar to those caused by mechanical injuries. As another example, in 1982 Steinman and coworkers described mice studies following pertussis immunization as follows:*

> *Post-mortem examination of the brain (in experimental mice) after immunization revealed diffuse vascular congestion and parenchymal haemorrhage in both the cortex and white matter. Cortical neurons showed ischaemic changes. Occasional areas of hypercellularity were evident in the meninges ... B pertussis has a wide range of physiological effects including increased IgE production, increased sensitivity to anaphylatic shock, lymphocytosis, and hyperinsulinaemia. Its ability to induce increased vascular permeability may account for the tendency to produce haemorrhage. (45)*
>
> *In terms of human studies, I have available a list of 109 references involving reports of adverse reactions from hepatitis B vaccine, a vaccine which appears to be especially prone to be followed by hemorrhagic complications. Among these reactions various forms of vasculitis (inflammation of blood vessels) appear with special frequency, which may contribute to hemorrhagic complications because of greater fragility and friability of blood vessels and consequently may mimic both cutaneous and cerebral hemorrhagic findings now considered to be diagnostic of **SBS**.*

It is also of concern that Drugs.com[152] mentions that in studies carried out on the Pentacel vaccine, four children died and others suffered bronchiolitis, dehydration, pneumonia, encephalopathy, and gastroenteritis within thirty days of vaccination. Of the children that died, special attention should be drawn to the fact that SIDS and head trauma were listed in the cause of death.

Serious Adverse Events

In Study P3T06, within 30 days following any of Doses 1-3 of Pentacel or Control vaccines, 19 of 484 (3.9%) participants who received Pentacel vaccine and 50 of 1,455 (3.4%) participants who received DAPTACEL + IPOL + ActHIB vaccines experienced a serious adverse event. Within 30 days following Dose 4 of Pentacel or Control vaccines, 5 of 431 (1.2%) participants who received Pentacel vaccine and 4 of 418 (1.0%) participants who received DAPTACEL + ActHIB vaccines experienced a serious adverse event. In Study 494-01, within 30 days following any of Doses 1-3 of Pentacel or Control vaccines, 23 of 2,506 (0.9%) participants who received Pentacel vaccine and 11 of 1,032 (1.1%) participants who received HCPDT + POLIOVAX + ActHIB vaccines experienced a serious adverse event. Within 30 days following Dose 4 of Pentacel or Control vaccines, 6 of 1,862 (0.3%) participants who received Pentacel vaccine and 2 of 739 (0.3%) participants who received HCPDT + POLIOVAX + ActHIB vaccines experienced a serious adverse event.

*Across Studies 494-01, 494-03 and P3T06, within 30 days following any of Doses 1-3 of Pentacel or Control vaccines, overall, the most frequently reported serious adverse events were bronchiolitis, dehydration, pneumonia and gastroenteritis. Across Studies 494-01, 494-03, 5A9908 and P3T06, within 30 days following Dose 4 of Pentacel or Control vaccines, overall, the most frequently reported serious adverse events were dehydration, gastroenteritis, **asthma,** and pneumonia.*

*Across Studies 494-01, 494-03, 5A9908 and P3T06, two cases of encephalopathy were reported, both in participants who had received Pentacel vaccine (N = 5,979). One case occurred 30 days post-vaccination and was secondary to cardiac arrest following cardiac surgery. One infant who had onset of neurologic symptoms 8 days post-vaccination was subsequently found to have structural cerebral abnormalities and was diagnosed with **congenital encephalopathy.***

A total of 5 deaths occurred during Studies 494-01, 494-03, 5A9908 and P3T06: 4 in children who had received Pentacel vaccine (N = 5,979) and one in a participant who had received DAPTACEL + IPOL + ActHIB vaccines (N = 1,455). There were no deaths reported in children who received HCPDT

*+ POLIOVAX + ActHIB vaccines (N = 1,032). Causes of death among children who received Pentacel vaccine were **asphyxia due to suffocation, head trauma, Sudden Infant Death syndrome,** and neuroblastoma (8, 23, 52 and 256 days post-vaccination, respectively). One participant with ependymoma died secondary to aspiration 222 days following DAPTACEL + IPOL + ActHIB vaccines."*

It is also worth considering the Pentacel information[152], as it clearly states in '*contraindications*' that

> **A severe allergic reaction (e.g., anaphylaxis) after a previous dose of Pentacel vaccine, any ingredient of this vaccine, or any other tetanus toxoid, diphtheria_toxoid, pertussis-containing vaccine, inactivated poliovirus vaccine or H influenzae type b vaccine is a contraindication to administration of Pentacel vaccine. (See Description). Because of uncertainty as to which ingredient of the vaccine may be responsible, none of the ingredients should be administered. Alternatively, such individuals may be referred to an allergist for evaluation if further immunizations are considered.**
>
> *The following events are contraindications to administration of any pertussis-containing vaccine, (19) including Pentacel vaccine.*
>
> **Encephalopathy (e.g., coma, decreased level of consciousness, prolonged seizures) within 7 days of a previous dose of a pertussis containing vaccine that is not attributable to another identifiable cause.**
>
> **Progressive neurologic disorder, including infantile spasms, uncontrolled epilepsy, progressive encephalopathy. Pertussis vaccine should not be administered to individuals with such conditions until the neurologic status is clarified and stabilized.**

It is all very well to state that these vaccines should not be given to an individual who is allergic to an ingredient; but if it is an infant's first dose in the two-months age group, no one knows how the infant will react or whether there will be a problem. It is also very unlikely that the doctor administering the vaccine or the parent will know if an infant has an allergy to any ingredient in the vaccine, especially if this is the child's first vaccine.

The patient information leaflet for Pediacel, another of the widely used five-in-one vaccines, is not much better.

> *Like all medicines, PEDIACEL can cause side effects, although not everybody gets them.*
> *Serious allergic reactions*
> ***If any of these symptoms occur after leaving the place where your child received his/her injection, you must consult a doctor IMMEDIATELY.*** *Serious allergic reactions are a very rare possibility (less than 1 in 10,000 children) after receiving any vaccine.*
> *These reactions may include:*
> *Difficulty in breathing, blueness of the tongue or lips, a rash, swelling of the face or throat, low blood pressure causing dizziness or collapse.*
> *When these signs or symptoms occur they usually develop quickly after the injection is given and while the child is still in the clinic or doctor's surgery.*
> *Other side effects*
> ***If your child experiences any of the following side effects and it gets serious or if you notice any side effects not listed in this leaflet, please tell your doctor, nurse or pharmacist.***
> *Very common reactions (reported in more than 1 in 10 children) are:*
> *Pain, redness and swelling at the injection site, irritability, decreased activity, fever (high temperature).*
> *Problems at the injection site are even more common when PEDIACEL is given as a booster vaccine.*
> *Common reactions (reported in less than 1 in 10 but more than 1 in 100 children) are:*
> *Loss of appetite, diarrhoea, being sick (vomiting).*
> *Rare reactions (reported in less than 1 in 1,000 but more than 1 in 10,000 children) are:*
> *a fit (convulsion) associated with a high temperature.*

Very rare reactions (reported in less than 1 in 10,000 children) are:

Abnormal crying, extensive limb swelling (from the injection site to beyond the joint).

Large injection site reactions (greater than 50 millimetres), including, extensive limb swelling from the injection site beyond one or both, joints may occur following vaccination with acellular Pertussis containing vaccines. These reactions start within 24-72 hours after vaccination, may be associated with redness, warmth, tenderness or pain at the injection site, and get better without the need for treatment within 3-5 days.

The following additional side effects have been reported during the commercial use of PEDIACEL:

Allergic reactions, hives, swollen face, a fit (convulsion) without a high temperature, high-pitched crying, a period of floppiness and decreased responsiveness that gets better without treatment and has no after effects, rash, pain in the vaccinated limb, high fever (temperature 40.5°C or higher)

injection site mass, paleness, feeling sleepy or drowsy (somnolence), tiredness or lack of energy (asthenia), lethargic (listlessness), rarely skin reactions have been reported that may include rashes (which may be itchy), swelling of the lower limbs, blueness, redness, severe crying and sometimes a purple, spotted rash of the legs that gets better without treatment.

My worry is that these vaccine information leaflets are in the vaccine boxes, so parents very rarely see them. Maybe if they did, then fewer children would have the serious adverse reactions that may lead to the neurological damage that can lead to the brain injuries that are occurring in cases of suspected SBS.

Michael D. Innis[153] says that he believes that vaccines can cause a vitamin C deficiency (Barlow's disease), especially if the mothers smoke and feed infants a formula-based feed. He says:

Apparent Life-Threatening Events (ALTEs), as defined by the National Institutes of Health, encompass all the findings hitherto attributed to Shaken Baby Syndrome (SBS), and may follow routine vaccination. Vaccines may also induce vitamin C deficiency (Barlow's disease), especially in formula-fed infants or infants whose mothers smoke. This could account for some of the changes seen in these infants, including hemorrhages, bruises, and fractures. Vitamin C deficiency should be excluded in patients suspected to have SBS.

He bases his paper on two cases where the children were said to have injuries caused by SBS. In his conclusion to his study, he said:

Although neither vitamin C levels nor histamine in the blood were measured, clinical, radiological, and laboratory findings suggest that the diagnosis of SBS should be questioned in these two cases. Poor nutrition and possible vaccine-induced vitamin C deficiency associated with temporary brittle bone disease may represent alternative explanations. Infantile scurvy, while uncommon in affluent countries, should nevertheless be routinely excluded before a diagnosis of SBS is made.

Both children in his study had had multiple vaccines just before their ALTE's had occurred, as is often the case in other studies carried out with children who have been said to have injuries consistent with being shaken. If many vaccines are given at one time, particularly if in multivaccine vials, then I see many more of these type of cases emerging.

Ingredients of the Five-in-One Vaccines

***Pentacel ingredients:*[154]**
Lyophilized Haemophilus b Conjugate Vaccine (bound to tetanus protein) -- Act HIB, and is to be reconstituted with Component Pertussis Vaccine and Deiphteria and Tetanus Toxoids Adsorbed combined with Inactivated Poliomyelitis Vaccine -- Quadracel.
Each .05 ml. dose of Act-HIB contains purified capsular polysaccharide covalently bound to tetanus protein .
Each .05 ml. dose of Quadracel contains pertussis toxoid, filamentous hemagglutinin, fimbriae, pertactin (a membrane protein), diphtheria toxoid, tetanus toxoid (inactivated with formaldehyde),

aluminium (.33mg), purified inactivated poliomyelitis vaccine: Type 1 (Mahoney); Type 2 (M.E.F.1); Type 3 (Saukett); and 0.6% + 0.1% added as preservative. The vaccine also contains 20 ppm <u>Tween</u> 80, less than 0.05% human albumin, and less than 1 ppm bovine serum. Trace amounts of polymyxin B and neomycin may be present from the cell growth medium. The three poliovirus types are inactivated by formalin (formaldehyde) and are grown on human diploid cells derived originally from aborted human fetuses. (Source: Compendium of Pharmaceuticals and Specialties 1999.)

PEDIARIX:[155]

PEDIARIX contains noninfectious proteins from diphtheria, tetanus, and pertussis bacteria, hepatitis B virus, and inactivated polio viruses. The vaccine also contains 2-phenoxyethanol (as a preservative), sodium chloride (NaCl), and aluminum salts. Low levels of formaldehyde, polysorbate 80, neomycin sulfate and polymyxin B (antibiotics), and yeast protein are present and thimerosal levels are undetectable. Manufactured by **GlaxoSmithKline Biologicals,** Rixensart, Belgium, Distributed by **GlaxoSmithKline,** Research Triangle Park, NC 27709.

PEDIACEL:[156]

Each 0.5 millilitre dose of PEDIACEL contains the following:
Active substances
Diphtheria Toxoid ....not less than 30 international units
Tetanus Toxoid ....not less than 40 international units
Acellular Pertussis Antigens
   Pertussis Toxoid ....20 micrograms
   Filamentous Haemagglutinin..................20 micrograms
   Pertactin (PRN................................ 3 micrograms
   Fimbriae types 2 and 3....................... 5 micrograms
Inactivated Poliomyelitis
   Type 1 (Mahoney ....40 D antigen units
   Type 2 (MEF-1 .... 8 D antigen units
   Type 3 (Saukett...........................32 D antigen units
Haemophilus influenzae Type b Polysaccharide
(Polyribosylribitol Phosphate....................10 micrograms
Conjugated to Tetanus Toxoid....................20 micrograms

Absorbed on Aluminium phosphate   1.5 milligrams (0.33 milligram Aluminium)

Other ingredients
2-phenoxyethanol, polysorbate 80 and water for injections.

Conclusion

The human infant brain has heightened vulnerability to inflammation due to its relatively high oxygen levels and high fat content, a large portion of which consists of polyunsaturated fatty acids, which are high in energetics but relatively unstable and susceptible to damaging peroxidation.

The Pourcyrous study, mentioned by Harold Buttram, MD, in Chapter 4, was the first of its kind and provides a unified theory of adverse vaccine reactions with documented brain inflammation, as indicated by increased levels of C-reactive protein in 70 percent of infants administered a single vaccine and 85 percent of those administered multiple vaccines; brain swelling (edema) would follow as one of the cardinal markers of inflammation; the brain swelling would immediately impact against the inner surface of the skull, cutting off (tourniquet-like) the passively outflowing of blood through the subdural venous network, this in turn resulting in a precipitous rise in intravenous venous pressure, the true cause of subdural hemorrhages in many of these cases in my opinion.

Very sadly, the potential protective role of antioxidants in these situations is being largely overlooked and ignored.

Many studies have shown that the vast majority of the children who die or suffer brain injuries thought to be an SBS/NAI event are not presenting any neck or spinal injuries. It has been shown from the studies presented by the neurosurgeon A. K. Ommaya, mentioned by Harold Buttram in Chapter 1, that infants who are shaken with the ferocity and violence required to inflict the type of injury associated with SBS should present evidence, to some degree at least, of neck or spinal injury. In many cases presented to the courts where SBS/NAI is suspected, the children have no external injuries whatsoever, and the evidence is purely based on neurological reporting alone.

It is very rare for a differential viewpoint to be considered or to be evidenced in court proceedings, particularly if the parent has reported that they suspect a vaccine injury may have occurred; and yet from the studies shown, there is a great deal of evidence to support the theory that vaccine injuries have caused children to die or have severe brain damage over many decades, especially surrounding multiple vaccines.

Each of the vaccines included in the five-in-one vaccine has a tainted history, with many hundreds of thousands of adverse reactions having been reported worldwide. These adverse reactions include encephalitis, convulsions (sometimes leading to epilepsy), uncontrollable screaming, exceptionally high temperatures, severe brain damage, and death. The common denominators linking all these vaccines are various chemicals and toxins, including thimerosal, aluminium, and formaldehyde, that are all known to be harmful to humans and other living creatures, causing various neurological conditions that are shown through the studies on rats and so on. It is worth repeating here that as scanners were not in full use until the mid to late 1970s, it would have been difficult to ascertain whether early accounts of high-pitched screaming, convulsions, and SID seen after vaccinations were, in fact, caused by undetected bleeds to the brain.

The five-in-one vaccine is given to infants from the age of two months, many of whom are premature. Due to the advances in medicine, babies are being saved at an earlier and earlier stage in their development, some being born at twenty-four weeks duration. This means that they could be vaccinated *before* the date they were meant to have been born. In reality, this means that they will be vaccinated with a dose of vaccine intended for a baby who is eight weeks old while they should still be in the womb. A full-term pregnancy should be forty weeks; a baby born at twenty-four weeks will be vaccinated at thirty-two weeks, which means they are actually *minus 8 weeks* when they are vaccinated.

Many babies born prematurely are sickly babies, often born with a variety of problems with a heightened risk of infection and respiratory problems. The problem is that these babies are actually targeted for vaccinations to protect them because they are seen as high risk. Timing for vaccinations is based on the age of a child from the day it is born; however, a premature baby is already at risk from bleeds to the brain or an intraventricular hemorrhage. It is clear from our evidence that many premature babies are presenting problems after routine vaccinations, including bleeds to the brain that are then identified as SBS. In my opinion, it is clear that the more vaccines that are being given to babies aged eight weeks old, the more parents are being falsely accused of SBS. It makes sense that the small, immature immune systems that young babies have cannot cope with a deadly combination of toxins and chemicals that are in our vaccines today.

All of which links back yet again to the Pourcyrous study, which highlights the fact that in premature babies in particular, **"intraventricular (brain) hemorrhages occurred in 17 percent of infants receiving single vaccines, with 24 percent incidence in those receiving multiple vaccines."** In our opinion, this is conclusive evidence showing that the more vaccines a premature baby in particular receives, the more chances there are for a bleed to the brain.

All in all, too many vaccines too early are proving to be extremely hazardous and are causing many parents worldwide to be falsely accused of SBS, particularly after their child has suffered a vaccine injury. Professionals involved in all aspects of child protection procedures must begin to be more open to a differential diagnosis as an alternative to the blame-the-parent theory.

References

(1) Schubert J, Riley EJ, Tyler SA. Combined effects in toxicology: A rapid systematic testing procedure: cadmium, mercury and lead. *Journal of Toxicology and Environmental Health,* 1978; 4:763-776.

(2) Abou-Donia MB, Wilmarth KR, Ochme F, Jensen KF, Kurt, TI. Neurotoxicity resulting from coexposure to pyridostigmine bromide, DEET, and permithrin: Implications of Gulf War chemical exposures. *Journal of Toxicology and Environmental Health, 1996; 48:35-56.*

(3) Arnold SF, Koltz DM, Collins B, Vonier PM, Guilette LJ, McLachlan JA. Synergistic activation of estrogen receptor with combinations of environmental chemicals. *Science,* 1996; 272: 1489-1492.

(4) Chester AC and Levine PH. Concurrent Sick Building Syndrome and Chronic Fatigue Syndrome: Epidemic Neuroalgia Revisited. *Clinical Infectious Disease,* 1994; 18(Suppl1): S43-8.

(5) Uscinski R. The Shaken Baby Syndrome. *J Amer Phys Surg.* Fall, 2004; 9(3):777.

(6) Ommaya AK. Whiplash injury and brain damage. *JAMA,* 1968; 204:75-79.

(7) Guthkelch A. Infantile subdural haematoma and its relationship to whiplash injuries. *BMJ,* 19712(759):430-431. http://www.pubmedcentral.nih.gov/articlerender.fegi?artid=1796151

(8) Caffey J. The parent-infant traumatic stress syndrome. *Am J Roentgen,* 1972;114:217-228.

(9) Caffey J. On the theory and practice of shaking infants. *Am J Dis Child,* 1972; 24:161-169.

(10) Caffey J. The whiplash shaken infant syndrome: Manual shaking by the extremities with whiplash-induced intracranial and intraocular pleadings, link with residual permanent brain damage and mental retardation. *Pediatrics,* 1974; 54:396-403.

(11) Bandak FA. Shaken Baby Syndrome: A biomechanics analysis of injury mechanisms, *Forensic Science Intern,* June 30, 2005; 151(1):71-79.

(12) Duhaime A-C, Gennarelli TA, Thibault LE, Bruce DA, Margulies SS, Wiser R. The shaken baby syndrome: a clinical, pathological and biomechanical study. *J Neurosurgery.* 1987; 66:409-15.

(13) Prange MT, Coats B, Raghupathi R, *et al.* Rotational loads during inflicted and accidental infant head injury. *J Neurosurgery.* 2001; Abst. D8; 18:1142.

(14) Ommaya AK, Goldsmith W, Thibault LE. Biomechanics and neuropathology of adult and paediatric head injury. *British J Neurosurgery.* 2002; 16:220-42.

(15) Prange MT, Coats B, Duhamie A-C, Margulies SS. Ahthropomorphic simulations of falls, shakes, and inflicted impacts in infants. *J Neurosurgery.* 2003; 99: 143-50.

(16) Goldsmith W, Plunkett J. A biomechanical analysis of the causes of traumatic brain injury in infants and children. *American J Forensic Med & Path.* 2004; 25:89-100.

(17) Bandak FA. Shaken baby syndrome: a biomechanics analysis of injury mechanisms. *Forensic Science Int.* 2005; 151151:71-79.

(18) Prang M, Newberry W, Moore T, Peterson D, Smyth B, Corrigan C. Inertial neck injuries in children involved in frontal collisions. SAE 2007 World Congress; Warrendale, PA; Society of Automotive Engineers; SAE paper #2007011170.

(19) Monson K, Sparrey C, Cheng L, Van Ee C, Manley G. Head exposure levels in pediatric falls. NNS 2007; abstract.

(20) Accessible on the internet under "Chris Van Ee Statement"

(21) Winter SCA, Quaghebeur G, Richards PG, Unusual cervical spine injury in a 1 year old, *Injury, International J. Care of Injured*, 2003; 34:316-391.

(22) Maguire S, Mann MK, Sibert J, Kemp A, Are there patterns of bruising in childhood which are diagnostic of Abuse? A systematic review, *Arch Dis Child*, 2005; 90:182-188.

(23) Plunkett J, Resuscitation injuries complicating the interpretation of premortem trauma and natural disease in children. *J Forens Sci*, 2006; 51(1):127-130.

(24) Hymel, KP, Jenny C, and Block, RW. Intracranial hemorrhage and rebleeding in suspected victims of abusive head trauma: addressing the forensic controversies. *Child Maltreatment.* 2002; 7(4):329-348.

(25) Plunkett, J. Fatal pediatric head injuries caused by short distance falls, *American Journal of Forensic Medicine and Pathology*, 2001; 22(1):1-12.

(26) Reiber, GD. Fatal falls in childhood, *American Juornal of Forensic Medicine and Pathology*, 1993; 14(3):201-207.

(27) Root, I. Head injuries from short distance falls, *American Journal of Forensic Medicine and Pathology*,1992; 13(1):83-87.

(28) *Nelson Textbook of Pediatrics,* 16th Edition, Behrman R.E., Kleigman, R.M., Jenson, H.B. (Editors), W.B. Saunders, 2000: page 489.

(29) Hayashi T, Hashimoto T, Fukuda S, Okudera T, and Ohsima Y.. Neonatal subdural hematoma secondary to birth injury. Clinical analysis of 48 survivors. *Child's Nervous System*, 1987; 3(1): 23-29.

(30) Hankins GD, Leight T, Van Hook J, Clark SL, Vines VL, Belfort MA. The role of forceps rotation in maternal and neonatal injury, *American Journal of Obstetrics and Gynecology,*1999; 180(1 Pt. 1):231-234.

(31) Hanigan, WC, Morgan, AM, Stahlberg, LK, Hiller JL.Tentorial hemorrhage associated with vacuum extraction, *Pediatrics,* 1990; 85(4): 534-539.

(32) Simonson C, Barlow P, Dehennin N, Sphel M, Toppet V, Murillo D., Neonatal complications of vacuum-assisted delivery. *Obstetrics & Gynecology,* 2007; 109(3):626-633.

(33) Castillo M, Fordham LA, MR of neurologically symptomatic newborns after vacuum extraction delivery, *Amer J Neuroradiology,* 1995; 16(4 Suppl.):816-818.

(34) Clark SL, Vines VL, Belfort MA, Fetal injury associated with routine vacuum use during cesarean delivery. *Amer. J. Obtetrics & Gynecology,* 2008,April; 198(4):e4. Epub 2008 Mar 4.

(35) Baume S, Cheret A, Creveuil C, Vardon D, Herlicoviez M, Dreyfus M. Complications of vacuum extractor deliveries. *Journal Gynecol ObstetBiol Reproduction,* (Paris) 2004; 33(4): 304-311.

(36) Piatt, JH, A pitfall in the diagnosis of child abuse: external hydrocephalus, subdural hematoma, and retinal hemorrhages. *Neurosurgery Focus,* 1999; 7(4), article 3:1-8.

(37) *Nelson Textbook of Pediatrics,* 16th Edition: page 489.

(38) Rutty, GN, Smith, CM, and Malia, RG. Late-form hemorrhagic disease of the newborn, *American Journal of Forensic Medicine and Pathology,* 1999; 20(1):48-51.

(39) Demiroren K, Yavuz H, Cam L, Intracranial hemorrhage due to vitamin K deficiency after the newborn period. *Pediatr Hematol Oncol,* 2004; 21(7):585-592.

(40) Parent, AD. Pediatric chronic subdural hematoma: A retrospective comparative analysis, *Pediatric Neurosurgery,* 1992; 18:266-271.

(41) Ito H, Yamamoto S, Komai T, Mizuboshi S, Fijisawa S, Kusiwaji S. Role of local hyperfibrinolysis in the etiology of chronic subdural hematoma, *Journal of Neurosurgery,* 1976; 45:26-31.

(42) Ito H, Komai T, Yamamoto S, Fibrinolytic enzyme in the lining walls of chronic subdural hematoma, *Journal of Neurosurgery,* 1978; 48:197-200.

(43) Ito H, Yamamoto S, Saito K, Quantitative estimation of hemorrhage in chronic subdural hematoma using the 51-Cr erythrocyte labeling method., *Journal of Neurosurgery,* 1987; 66:862-864.

(44) Kalokerinos A. *Medical Pioneer of the 20th Century, an Autobiography.* Melbourne, Australia, Biology Therapies Publishing, 2000: 11-26.

(45) Clemetson CAB. *Vitamin C,* Volumes I, II, & III. CRC Press, Boca Raton, 1989.

(46) Hume R, Weyers E. Changes in the leucocyte ascorbic acid concentration during the common cold. *Scot Med J,* 1973; 18:3.

(47) Clemetson CAB. Barlow's Disease, *Medical Hypothesis.* 2002; 59(1):52-56.

(48) Doughty LA, Nguyen KB, Durbin JE, and Biron CA. A role for IFN-Alpha Beta in virus infection-induced sensitization to endotoxin. *Journal of Immunology,* 2001; 166:2658-2664.

(49)Johnston DS, Thompson MS. Vitamin C status of an out-patient population. *American J Clinical Nutrition,* 1998; 17:366-370.

(50) Clemetson, CAB. Histamine and ascorbic acid in human blood. *Journal of Nutrition,* 1980; 110:662-668.

(51) Chaterjee JB, Majunder AK, Nandi BK, Subramanian N. Synthesis and some major functions of vitamin C in animals, *Annals New york Academy of Science,* 1975; 258:24-47.

(52) Dey, PK. Efficacy of vitamin C in counteracting tetanus toxin toxicity, *Naturwissenschaften,* 1966; 53:319.

(53) Jungblut CW, Zweemer RL. Inactivation of diphtheria toxin in vivo and in vitro by crystalline vitamin C (ascorbic acid), *Proceedings of the Society of Experimental Biology & Medicine,* 1935; 32:1229-1234.

(54) Gore I, Tanaka Y, Fujinami T, Shirahama T. Endothelial changes produced by ascorbic acid deficiency in guinea pigs. *Arch Pathology,* 1965; 80:371-376.

(55) Barlow T. On cases described as 'acute rickets,' which are probably a combination of scurvy and rickets; the scurvy being an essential and rickets being a variable element. *Med Chir Trans,* 1883; 66:159.

(56) Hart C, Lessing O. *Der Scorbut der Kleinen Kinder (Moller-barlowsche Krankheit).* Stuttgart: Verlag von Ferdinand Enke, 1913.

(57) O'Brien JS. Stability of the myelin membrane; *Science.* 1965; 147:1099-1107.

(58) Stocker JT, Dehner LP. Eds, *Pediatric Pathology,* Vol. 2, Philadelphia, PA.: Lippincott Williams & Wilkins, 2002:1449.

(59) Nolty J. *The Human Brain, an Introduction to Its Functional Anatomy.* Fifth Edition, Mosby Publ, Philadelphia, PA:129.

(60) Yavin E, Brand A, Green P. Docosahexanenoic acid abundance in the brain: a biodevice to combat oxidative stress. *Nutr Neurosci,* 2002; 5(3):149-157.

(61) Cunnane SC, Francescutti V, Brenna T, Crawford MA. Breast-

fed infants achieve a higher rate of brain and whole body docosa-hexanenoate accumulation than formula-fed infants not consuming dietary docosahexaenoate. *Lipids,* 2000; 35(1):1-5-111.

(62) Innis SM. The role of dietary n-6 and n-3 fatty acids in the developing brain. *Devel Neurosci,* 2000; 22(5-6):474-480.

(63) Crawford MA, Bloom M, Cunnane S, Holmsen H, Ghebremeskel, Schmidt, WS. Docosahexanenoic acid and cerebral evolution. *World Rev Nutr Diet,* 2001; 88:6-17.

(64) Yavin ES, Glozman S, Green PN, Cunnane SC. Docosahexaenoic acid accumulation in the prenatal brain: prooxidant and antioxidant features. *J Mol Neurosci,* 2001, 16(2-3):229-235:279-284.

(65) Larque EH, Demmelmair H, Koletzko B. Perinatal supply and metabolism of long-chain polyunsaturated fatty acids; importance for the early development of the nervous system. *Ann NY Acad Sci,* 2002; 967:299-310.

(66) Haynes RI, Borenstein NS, Desilva TM, Folkerth RD, Liu LG, Volpe JJ, Kinney HC. Axonal development in the cerebral white matter of the human fetus and infant. *Journal of ComparativeNeurology,* 2005; 484:156-167.

(67) Tauscher MK, Berg D, Brockmann M, Seiden-Spinner S, Speer CP, Vollard E. Association of histologic chorioamnionitis: Increased levels of cord blood cytokines, and intracerebral hemorrhage in preterm neonates. *Bio Neonate,* 2003; 83:166-170.

(68) *Maternal-Fetal Medicine, Principles and Practice.* Creasy RK, Reznik R Editors, Philadelphia: W.B. Saunders, 1994:1169.

(69) Whitby EH, Griffiths PD, Rutter S, Smith H, Sprigg A, Ohadike P *et al.* Frequency and natural history of subdural haemorrhages in babies and relation to obstetric factors. *Lancet,* 2004; 8:363:846-851.

(70) Rooks, VJ, Eaton, JP, Ruess, L, Petermann GW, Keck-Wherley J,

Pedersen RC. Prevalence and evolution of intracranial hemorrhage in asymptomatic term infants. *American Society of Neuroradiology, American Journal Neuroradiology,* 2008; www.ajnr.org

(71) *Forensic Pathology, Principles and Practice,* Dolinak D, Matshes E, Lew E. Elsevier Academic Press, New York, 2005: 431-435.

(72) Rensburg, SJ van, Zyl J van, Hon D, Daniels W, Hendricks J, Potoknic F, *et al.* Biochemical Model for Inflammation of the Brain: the effect of iron and transferrin on monocytes and lipid peroxidation. *Metabolic Brain Disease,* 2004; 19(1/2):97-112.

(73) Sen S, Cloete Y, Hassan K, Buss P, Adverse events following vaccination in premature infants, *Acta Paediatr,* 2001; 33(5):418-421.

(74) Sanchez PJ, Laptook AR, Fisher L *et al* Apnea after immunization of preterm infants, *J Pediatr,* `1997; 130(5):746-751.

(75) Slack MH, Schapira D. Severe apneas following immunization in premature infants, *Archives Dis Child Fetal Neonatal Ed,* 1999; 81(1):F67-68.

(76) Pourcyrous M, Korones SB, Kristopher LA, and Bada HS. Primary immunization of premature infants with gestational age <35 weeks: Cardiorespiratory complications and C-reactive protein responses associated with administration of single and multiple separate vaccines simultaneously. *J Pediatr,* 2007; 151:167-172.

(77) Iwasa S, Ishida S, Akama K. Swelling of the brain caused by pertussis vaccine: its quantitative determination and the responsible factors in the vaccine, *Japan J Med Sci Biol,* 1985; 38(2):53-65.

(78) Levine S. Hyperacute encephalomyelitis, *Amer J Pathol,* 1973. 37:247-250.

(79) Munoz JJ, Bernard CE, Mackay IR. Elicitation of experimental encephalomyelitis in mice with aid of pertussigen, *Cellular Immunol.*1984; 83:92-100.

(80) Squier W, Mack J. The neuropathology of infant subdural hemorrhages. *Forensic Science International,* in press, doi:10.1016/j. forsciint.2009.02.005.

(81) Orlin JR, Osen KK, Hovig T. Subdural compartment in pig: A morphologic study with blood and horseradish peroxidase infused subdurally. *Anatomic Research,* 1991; 230(1): 22-37.

(82) Blaylock, RI. The danger of excessive vaccination during brain development. *Medical Veritas.* 2008; April, 5(1): 1727-1741.

(83) Blaylock, RI. Chronic microglial activation and excitotoxicity secondary to excessive immune stimulation: possible factors in Gulf War Syndrome and autism. *Journal American Physians and Surgeons,* 2004; 9(2):46-52.

(84) Blaylock RI. The danger of excessive vaccination during brain development: the case for a link to Autism Spectrum Disorders (ASD). *Medical Veritas,* 2008; 1727-1741.

(85) King PG. Thimerosal in vaccines: Inconvenient reality. *Medical Veritas,* 2008; 5(2): 1816-1820.

(86) Fraser, Heather, The History of the Peanut Allergy, First Published in Canada by Espresso Book Machine, McMaster University Innovative Press, Hamilton, Ontario, 2010.

(87) Romansky MJ, Rittman GE, A method of prolonging the action of penicillin, *Science,* Sept. 1st, 1944; 196-198.

(88) Jones, SW, Peanut oil used in new vaccine; product patented for Merck said to extend immunity, *New York Times, Business-Financial Section,* Sept. 19, 1954; 31. (89) Smith, JWG, Response to influenza vaccine in adjuvant 65-4. *Journal of Hygiene,* 1974; 74(2): 251-259.

(90) http://www.patentstorm.us/patents/6299884/description. html;

(91) P. Gecher (Ed.), *Encyclopedia of Emulsion Technology:Applications* (Marcel Dekker, 1985), 191.

(92) Allison AC, Byars NE, Immunoogical adjuvants: general properties and side effects, *Mol. Immunol,* 1991; 28(3): 279-284.

(93) Langmuir AD, An epidemiologic and clinical evaluation of Guillan-Barre Syndrome reported in association with the administration of Swine influenza vaccines. *American Journal of Epidemiology,* 1984; 119(6):841-879.

(94) Barnum AM, Lukacs SL. Food allergy among U.S. children. Trends and prevalence in hospitalizations. *National Centre for Health Statistics* CDC, (Oct. 22, 2008).

(95) Bock SA, Furlong AM, Sampson HA. Fatalities due to anaphylactic reactions to food. *Journal of Allergy and Clinical Immun,* Jan. 2001; 107(1):191-193.

(96) Ford ES, Liu S, Mannino DM, Giles WH, Smith SJ. C-Reactive protein concentration and concentrations of blood vitamins, carotenoids, and selenium among United States adults. *Europ. J.Clin. Nutr.* 2003; 57:1157-1163.

(97) Wannamethee SG, Lowe GDO, Rumley A, Bruckdorfer KR, Whincup PH. Association of vitamin C status, fruit and vegetable intakes, and markers of inflammation and hemostasis. *Am J. Clin. Nutri.,* 2006; 83:567-574.

(98) Romagnani S. Biology of TH1 and TH2 cells. *Journal of Clinical Immunology,* 1995; 15(3):121-29.

(99) Wakefield AJ, Murch SH, Anthony A, Linnell J, Cassen DM, Malik M, *et al.* Heal-nodular hyperplasia, non-specific colitis, and pervasive developmental disorder in children. *Lancet,* 1998; 351:637-41.

(100) Wakefield AJ, Anthony A, Murch SH, Thomson MA, Montgomery SM, Davies S *et al. Am J Gastroenterology,* 2000; 95(9):2285-2295.

(101) Uhlman V, Martin CM, Pilkington I, Silva I, Killalea A, Murch SB, Wakefield AJ, O'Leary JJ. Potential viral pathogenic mechanism for new varian inflammatory bowel disease. *J Clin Path & Molecular Path,* 2002; 55:0-6.

(102) Sources: Centers for Disease Control and Prevention, California Department of Health and Human Services.

(103) Miller NZ. *Vaccine Safety Manual,* 2008; Sante Fe, NM: New Atlantean Press, Page 202

(104) Jahnke U. Sequence homology between certain viral proteins and proteins related to encephalomyelitis and neuritis. *Science,* 1985; 29:242-284.

(105) Brody JA, Overfield T, Mammes IM. Depression of tuberculin reaction by viral (measles) vaccines. *New England Journal of Medicine,* 1964; 711:1294-1296.

(106) Karp C, Wysocka M, Wakefield AJ *et al.* Mechanism of suppression of cell-mediated immunity by measles virus. *Science,* 1996; 273:228-231.

(107) Kerdiles YM, Sellin CI, Druelle J, Horvat B. Immunosuppression by measles virus: role of viral proteins. *Rev Medical Virology,* 2006; 16:49-63.

(108) Fraser, Heather, The History of the Peanut Allergy, First Published in Canada by Espresso Book Machine, McMaster University Innovative Press, Hamilton, Ontario, 2010.

(109) Romansky MJ, Rittman GE, A method of prolonging the action of penicillin, *Science,* Sept. 1st, 1944; 196-198.

(110) Jones, SW, Peanut oil used in new vaccine; product patented for Merck said to extend immunity, *New York Times, Business-Financial Section,* Sept. 19, 1954; 31.

(111) Smith, JWG, Response to influenza vaccine in adjuvant 65-4. *Journal of Hygiene,* 1974; 74(2): 251-259.

(112) http://www.patentstorm.us/patents/6299884/description. html;

(113) P. Gecher (Ed.), *Encyclopedia of Emulsion Technology:Applications* (Marcel Dekker, 1985), 191.

(114) Allison AC, Byars NE, Immunoogical adjuvants: general properties and side effects, *Mol. Immunol,* 1991; 28(3): 279-284.

(115) Langmuir AD, An epidemiologic and clinical evaluation of Guillan-Barre Syndrome reported in association with the administration of Swine influenza vaccines. *American Journal of Epidemiology,* 1984; 119(6):841-879.

(116) Barnum AM, Lukacs SL. Food allergy among U.S. children. Trends and prevalence in hospitalizations. *National Centre for Health Statistics* CDC, (Oct. 22, 2008).

(117) Bock SA, Furlong AM, Sampson HA. Fatalities due to anaphylactic reactions to food. *Journal of Allergy and Clinical Immun,* Jan. 2001; 107(1):191-193.

(118) England, Christina, 5-in-1 Vaccines, publication pending.

(119) http://www.autism-end-it-now.org/

(120) Al-Bayati MA, Analysis of causes that led to baby Jackie Ray's developmental delay and intracranial bleeding. *Medical Veritas,* 2008; Vol. 5 (2).

(121) Al-Bayati MA, Analysis of causes that led to baby Ryan's hemorrhagic pneumonia, cardiac arrest, intracranial bleeding, and retinal bleeding. *Medical Veritas,*2008; Vol. 5 (2).

(122) Al-Bayati MA. Analysis of causes that led to baby Huda Sharif's

intracranial and retinal bleeding and fractures of the left humerus and the 7th rib. *Medical Veritas,* 2009; Vol 6 (1).

(123) Stewart Professor G.T. Infectivity and virulence of tubercle bacilli." Lancet 2; 562 . http://www.whale.to/vaccines/stewart1. html

(124) Stewart, Professor G. T. Toxicity of Pertussis Vaccine: Frequency and Probability of Adverse Reactions, *Journal of Epidemiology & Community Health* 33 (1979):150–156.

(125) Fox Rosemary, Commission Europeenne Des Droits De L'Homme European Commission of Human Rights Application Form, "The Association of Parents of Vaccine Damaged Children—Case for Compensation for Vaccine Damaged Children," August 9, 1975.

(126) Coulter Harris L., PhD, SIDS and Seizures, 1982.http://www. whale.to/v/coulter1.html

(127) Baraff L. J. et al., "Possible Temporal Association Between Diphtheria-Tetanus Toxoid-Pertussis Vaccination and Sudden Infant Death Syndrome, *Pediatric Infectious Disease Journal* 1983 Jan–Feb;2(1):7–11.

(128) Gaublomme Kris, MD, "Acellular Pertussis—The International Vaccination," Newsletter March 1998.

(129) Blakemore-Brown Lisa, Psychologist, "Cot Deaths and Vaccines—Child Protection Turned on Its Head, Thimerosal Thoughts," http://thimerosalthoughts-bb.blogspot.com/2007/08/ cot-deaths-and-vaccines-child.html.

(130) The National Vaccine Information Centre (NVIC) Haemophilus Influenza Type B Vaccine (HIB) http://www.nvic.org/Vaccines-and-Diseases/HIB.aspx

(131) Encephalitis Society *website* http://www.encephalitis.info/

(132) Winkler, Dawn "Vaccine Ingredients and Contact Info," http://

www.tetrahedron.org/articles/vaccine_awareness/ingredients.
html.

(133) White Heidi, Hospital Pharmacist, "Can Hib Vaccine Cause
Asthma?" http://www.whale.to/vaccines/hib2.html.

(134) DiMiceli Lauren et al., "Vaccination of Yeast Sensitive
Individuals: Review of Safety Data in the U.S. Vaccine Adverse
Event Reporting System (VAERS)," *Science Direct* 2006 http://
www.sciencedirect.com/science?_ob=ArticleURL&_udi=B6TD4-
4GV2PDP-6&_user=10&_coverDate=02%2F06%2F2006&_
rdoc=1&_fmt=high&_orig=search&_origin=search&_
sort=d&_docanchor=&view=c&_searchStrId=1527405295&_
rerunOrigin=google&_acct=C000050221&_version=1&_urlVer-
sion=0&_userid=10&md5=dab143480aae9e3cc754480e04c83e5
c&searchtype=a .

(135) Scheibner Viera, PhD, "Shaken Baby Syndrome: The
Vaccination Link," from *Nexus* Aug.–Sept. 1998, http://www.whale.
to/vaccines/sbs.html.

(136) Rense.com http://www.rense.com/general59/vvac.htm

(137) Maybury Okonek Bonnie A. and Morganstein Linda, editor,
Development of Polio Vaccines, Access Excellence Classic Collection
http://www.accessexcellence.org/AE/AEC/CC/polio.php .

(138) McBean,Eleanor , The Poisoned Needle – Suppressed Facts
About Vaccination 1957 Chapter 10 Hidden Dangers of the Polio
Vaccine http://www.whale.to/a/mcbean5.html.

(139) Mclean, Louise LCCH, MARH, "Shaken Baby Syndrome
2004,"http://www.thenhf.com/vaccinations_18.htm.

(140) Rense.com as above http://www.rense.com/general59/vvac.
htm

(141) Damato, Dr. Gregory PhD, citizen journalist, "Hepatitis B
Vaccine: Good for 'Newborn' Prostitutes and Drug Users, but Who

Else?" **Natural News**, July 11, 2008, http://www.naturalnews.com/023610_hepatitis_B_vaccination.html.

(142) BioPharm International, "Recombinant Vaccine Production in Yeast," http://biopharminternational.findpharma.com/biopharm/Downstream+Processing/Recombinant-Vaccine-Production-in-Yeast/ArticleStandard/Article/detail/485189.

(143) The Hepatitis B Foundation http://www.hepb.org/hepb/vaccine_information.htm

(144) CBS News report, "Court Links Hepatitis B Vaccine to a Death," Feb. 2, 2009, http://www.cbsnews.com/8301-501263_162-4770907-501263.html.

(145) England Christina, "Another Vaccine, Another Lie, Another Day in Government," *American Chronicle,* April 14, 2009, http://www.americanchronicle.com/articles/view/98286.

(146) Girard Dr Marc Autoimmun Rev 2005; 4: 96–100

(147) Alternatives to Vaccines Made from Aborted Babies," Catherine Williams http://www.dgwsoft.co.uk/homepages/vaccines/alternatives.htm

(148) The Deccan Herald http://www.deccanherald.com/content/84618/five-one-vaccine-led-child.html

(149) LankaNewspapers.com, "Five-in-One Vaccine Led to Child Deaths in Sri Lanka—BMJ, July 30, 2010, http://www.lankanewspapers.com/news/2010/7/58942.html.

(150) West Edda from VRAN, http://www.whale.to/a/west5.html.

(151) Buttram Harold E. MD, "Shaken Baby/Impact Syndrome: Flawed Concepts and Misdiagnoses" (based on a review of 22 cases). http://www.woodmed.com/Shaken%20Baby%20Web%202002.htm

(152) Drugs.com http://www.drugs.com/pro/pentacel.html

(153) Innis Dr. Michael D., MBBS, "Vaccines, Apparent Life-Threatening Events, Barlow's Disease, and Questions about Shaken Baby Syndrome." **Journal of American Physicians and Surgeons Volume 11 Number 1 Spring 2006**(154) Pentacel **Pentacel/ Pediacel** vaccine notes and ingredients http://www.whale.to/v/pentacel.html

(155) Pedarix Patient Information, http://www.scotlandcounty-health.org/docs/Pediarix.pdf.

(156) Piadacel Patient information leaflet, available in pdf format at http://www.medicines.org.uk/emc/medicine/17468/PIL/PEDIACEL/.

About the Authors

Harold E Buttram, MD

In January 2009 Dr. Buttram retired from medical practice after 50 years of work in the fields of family practice and environmental medicine. In the latter years of practice he treated many children with autism and related disorders as a referral physician for the Autism Research Institute (ARI). At one of the ARI conferences in the 1990s, Bernard Rimland, Ph.D., founding director of ARI, announced that in over half of the autistic children seen by ARI referral physicians, formerly normal children had abruptly and dramatically regressed into autism in a time-related fashion following the MMR vaccine. On learning this, Dr. Buttram checked on his own computerized medical records and found similar patterns in the autistic children in his practice.

This also coincided with a time period in which Dr. Buttram had become involved as a defense witness in Shaken Baby Syndrome (SBS) cases, so that he began checking for a time-based relationship between symptoms and radiological findings of subdural (brain) hemorrhages (on which almost all charges of SBS were based) and routine vaccinations. In most instances, such a relationship was clearly evident. However, in those early years there was little proof that would stand up in court, so that it was usually wise to turn to other medical issues for defense.

This has now dramatically changed. In 2007 a study involving 239 preterm infants was performed in which C-Reactive Protein blood tests (a standard blood test marker for inflammation) was performed on 239 preterm infants who received either a single vaccine or mixed vaccines in a pediatric intensive care unit (Pourcyrous *et al. Journal Pediatrics,* 2007). The first definitive study of its kind, it provided a unified theory of adverse vaccine reactions and their pathogenesis, as reviewed in this text.

Christina England

Christina was born and educated in London, U.K. She left school to work in a children's library, specializing in story telling and book buying. In 1978 Christina changed her career path to dedicate her time to caring for the elderly and was awarded the title of *Care Giver of the Year* for her work with the elderly in 1980.

After dedicating much of her spare time helping disabled children in a special school, she then worked in a respite unit in a leading teaching hospital.

In 1990 Christina adopted the first of two disabled boys, both with challenging behavior, complex disabilities, and medical needs. In 1999 she was accused of *Munchausen by Proxy* after many failed attempts to get the boys' complex needs met. Finally, she was cleared of all accusations after an independent psychologist gave both boys the diagnosis of Autism Spectrum Disorder and ADHD as part of a complex tapestry of disorders. During the assessments it was discovered through the foster care diaries that the eldest boy had reacted adversely to the MMR vaccine.

After taking *A Level* in Psychology and a *BTEC* in Learning Disabilities Ms. England then spent many years researching vaccines and adverse reactions. She went on to gain an HND in journalism and media and is currently writing for the *American Chronicle*, the *Weekly Blitz* and *Vaccination Truth* on immunization safety and efficacy.

England's main area of expertise is in researching the areas surrounding false allegations of child abuse. Her work is now read internationally and has been translated into many languages. England has been a guest on *Holy Hormones Honey – The Greatest Story Never Told!* on KRFC FM 88.9 in, Colorado. She speaks at seminars worldwide and has been invited to speak in London and Canada in 2011.